C000164475

Rapid Weight Loss Hypnosis

Ultimate and powerful guide to lose weight fast and naturally through daily meditation, affirmation, mini-habits, and self-esteem.

By

Jodie K. Hunt

CONTENTS

INTRODUCTION

Hypnosis may be defined as a routine causing an alternate state of awareness, which assists people to end up being extremely sensitive to a hypnotherapist's recommendations.

This routine has been accepted in psychoanalysis for treating psychic health problems by revisiting the hazardous events they experienced in the past (specifically during childhood) and then by transmitting recommendations developed to help them.

Itmight be utilized to reduce stress or tension. Hypnosis may help you remain calm before a huge test and during your big speech.

Hypnosis might control blood circulation and different autonomic functions that are not generally based on conscious adjustment. The relaxing reaction that occurs with hypnosis also modifies the neurohormonal systems that control many body functions.

For weight-loss, it might help you to pass when everything else has actually failed. Using hypnosis, we may help you achieve the weight-loss that you want. Hypnosis may go straight to the centerof the issue and focus on changing particular habits or routines with healthy options.

Itmight likewise be used to change those who suffer from anxiety attacks. These are categorized by the incapacity to focus, problems in making decisions, severe sensitivity, disharmony, sleep interruptions, extreme sweating, and consistent muscle stress.

Hypnosis may aid by giving you coping systems so that whenever tension causing circumstances to take place, you are able to face them withbetter-suited methods. Itmight be utilized in lots of numerous ways.

Hypnosis might likewise be a technique of pain control, typically utilized with burn victims and ladies in labor. Itcannot depose an exercise routinebut might carry out and enhance it.

Hypnotic affirmations have a cumulative healing effect in the subconscious part of the mind, with the ability to enhance a healthy self-esteem. Hypnosis can't make an individual do anything against their will or that opposes their worths.

A hypnotherapist has principles thatare requiredto develop just those changes that abide by agreed-upon framework.

Hypnosis cannot just help you to get individual achievements, however,it can help you stay determined towards achievingthose objectives. After a few sessions of "hypnosis therapy," you might find more desire in living, and have more energy than ever pictured.

Some of the additional benefits of using hypnosis for weight reduction include:

1. Improved sleep.

2. An overall feeling of wellbeing.

3. The release of endorphins and other feel-good chemicals in the brain.

4. Improved self-confidence.

5. Increased immune system efficiency

6. Reduction in stress levels.

Do not get yourself worried too much. If you do try hypnosis for weight reduction you will loseweight. Something that you have to bear in mind is hypnosis for weight-loss is not a magic tablet. You will still need to wish to loseweight and it will still take your will power. You require to follow the hypnosis for weight-loss program you select and stay with it. If you do these simple things you can be on your way to a better, slimmer you. Let's read further on some SELF-HELP HYPNOSIS FOR WEIGHT LOSS

However, the truth is that no one really can blame you if you think it could be a lie. I bet you should have got the basics of self-help hypnosis by now; hypnosis and subliminal messages, I hope. I'm not sure about you, but I had the opportunity to watch a magician put his volunteer in a trance. All the magicians did was repeat somesentences.

Okay, self-hypnosis works like this. The only difference you need to know is that self-hypnosis is certainly not brainwashing. You will use hypnosis to change your thinking. In this scenario, it aims to change the way weight loss is dealt with.

Using Self Hypnosis

Everyone will lose some weight for a few weeks or months before the old temptations reemerge. Yet this must not be the way! You can use the power of self-hypnosis to lose weight.

There are many different food plans to choose from, and the same is true with self-hypnosis for weight loss. You may complain that the virtual shelf is groaning under the weight of many books about weight loss, but it means that regardless of why you're trying to lose weight, there is a specially written hypnosis product waiting for you.

So, what separates self-hypnosis from using willpower?

Although willpower works with your conscious mind, self-hypnosis deepens: down into the unconscious part of your mind, the part which most of the time controls what you do. It regulates stuff like breathing, pumping blood throughout the body, and many other things we take for granted.

It also tracks our understanding of food. Food has traditionally been scarce. We are, therefore, conditioned to use the periods when food is plentiful. That means almost 24 hours a day, seven days a week in today's modern society.

Self-hypnosis for weight loss can work to teach the unconscious mind to know that whenever you want, you should eat. You'll start to see the change of attitude with hardly any effort on your part, and you will be able to try all those beautiful clothes you felt you had to throw away because they no longer fit.

Self-Hypnosis For Weight Loss – Four Easy Steps

You may think of someone lying on a sofa being spokento ina soothing voice, or perhaps it's one of those old TV shows where a bright and slow watch hypothesizes someone, while it can be that hundreds of thousands of people around the world practice self-hypnosis for weight loss and it is highly effective when done correctly.

Self-hypnosis is quite easy to use for weight loss. You are using methods such as visualization and positive self-talk to train your mind to think in a new way when your body is completely relaxed.

Step 1: the first thing to do is to get comfortable with self-hypnosis for weight loss. Sitting downwould work best; just make sure you don't fall asleep. To release stress in your body, tense and relax every part of your body, from your forehead to your feet. You can envision this while standing under a gentle waterfall and imagine that the water that flows through your body washes all your tension.

Step 2:you'll want to focus on your breathing next. Imagine that fresh oxygen fills your body if you inhale clean air. When you exhale slowly, your body relaxes. To deepen your sense of relaxation, you should imagine yourself slowly going down a long escalator or simply count down to100 while you focus on calming your body.

STEP 3:once you're completely relaxed, you'll use positive statements to solve your problems. If you use self-hypnosis in weight loss, you might want to discover ideas such as "I enjoy the taste of fruits and vegetables," "I love how I look after workouts," or "I enjoy being slim and healthy."

STEP 4: to return to consciousness, just count from zeroto 10 as you concentrate on numbers until you feel completely awake. You may have to count more than once from zeroto 10 until you are ready to start normal activities again.

Developing your own weight loss hypnosis plan will help you finally overcome barriers that prevent you from losing weight.

How Do I Make Hypnosis Work For Weight Loss?

Self-help weight loss hypnosis operates by using subliminal messages. For so many years, subliminalmessages have been the focus of study, actually since the 19th century.

Such messages will be conveyedin various ways. Sounds, pictures, and sentences are like that. The subliminal messages are the kind of messages that don't move through your mind and process data through reason or logic.

Alternatively, subliminal messages go straight to your subconscious mind, which is not entirely controlled by you. As a consequence, the messages are generally not filtered and are simply accepted by your subconscious.

What are subliminalmessages, and what do they do to achieve weight loss?

In the event of self-hypnosis for weight loss, subliminal messages are usually called statements. These are positive statements that should lift you and help you to overcome this challenge.

These positive statements must be repeated many times to ensure that they pass through your unconscious mind, and without even thinking about them, you can keep these optimistic declarations in mind. The body tends to practice these convictions.You're going to feel starving. You'll be picky about the food you eat. In several strenuous activities, you have more energy and vitality to interact and are also less depressed and anxious about your struggles.

Tactics Complementing Weight Loss Hypnosis

Have you purchased mp3s and CDs to help you quickly receive your subliminal messages for your weight loss? The tracks often include incredibly soothing, repeated words accompanied by instrumental music. You just have to listen to the tracks.

Are there weight loss disadvantages to self-help hypnosis?

If you don't follow the tips, you can't gain as much from self-help hypnosis. It is worth often doing so that the subconscious thoughts can receive subliminal messages and assimilate them.

Besides, you must be hypnotized without distractions. Therefore, you should get into a relaxed and peaceful environment before taking part in a session. Clear your mindfrom meaningless thoughts, too.

Some of the potential benefits of weight reduction hypnosis include.

1. Lower stress rate.

2. Better night's sleep.

3. Endorphins and other chemicals are released in the brain.

4. Increased performance of the immune system

5. Improved self-confidence.

6. An overall sense of well-being.

Looking at overall hypnosis is excellent even if you don't lose any weight. Don't worry; you're going to lose weight if you try hypnosis for weight loss. One thing you must know is weight loss is not a magic pill. You still have to lose weight, and some of your will power will always be taken. You have to obey the weight loss system hypnosis that you choose to live with. You can be on the way to a healthier, slimmer body if you do those simple things.

Hypnosis (state theory) is a state of mind or collection of behaviors (non-state theory) usually caused by a technique known as a hypnotic induction, normally consisting of a series of preliminary guidelines and ideas.

Hypnosis and self-hypnosis are now being used for many reasons. The practice is not yet quite widespread, and many are embracing the idea as well.

Strictly speaking, nobody says you can't let pounds disappear, as though by chance, by means ofhypnosis. Yes, hypnosis is intended to reprogram the subconscious mind to be different. After all, your acts and many other facets of your physical health have to do with your weight. So, it doesn't seem so difficult to believe.

So, what kind of changes in our actions can hypnosis cause?

- Eat fewer calories
- Eat healthier–allow better shopping/cooking/ordering choices
- Exercise More–more energy when exercising
- Better self-image–minimize self-sabotage

Would hypnosis really do these things?

In theory, indeed. Does everybody who tries it always get good results? Regrettably, no. But nothing works for all, like diets, exercise or diet pills.

Nonetheless, what is hypnosis?

"Hypnosis" is a relatively new term that was invented by a man from the 19th century, named Franz Mesmer (from whom the word "mesmerism" means necessarily the same thing as hypnosis). It means entering a state of trance where you are highly suggestible. Recently, scientists have identifiedspecific brain waves that occur during these conditions.

Initially, hypnosis was synonymous with stage hypnotics and magicians who would make people under hypnosis do entertaining and weird stuff. Nevertheless, it was also used for therapeutic purposes at the same time. It fits into the evolving psychological field, which emphasizes the role of the subconscious mind in our actions.

Types of Hypnosis

There are many ideas and hypotheses concerning hypnosis, but we're only going to look at two main types in this relatively short document. One is clinicalhypnosis, done by a hypnotist or a hypnotherapist. The other is self-hypnosis, which is more like sleep when you relax and goo into a trance.

One of the most popular types of self-hypnosis today is the use of technology to create a trance. This is typically a recording of relaxing music that can also includesuggestions that have a positive influence. Prosperity, better health, confidence, and, of course, weight loss are noted.

Some hypnosis tape, CDs, or MP3s use subliminal messages that some scientists find makes the subconscious mind more efficient. Others use what are called binaural beats, where different frequencies are used in each ear (to align the two hemispheres of the brain, you need headphones for this effect).

Using Hypnosis For Weight Loss

How would you like to lose weight with hypnosis? Okay, a trained hypnotherapist could be visited. Although this is not inexpensive, compared to any form of traditional therapy, it has the advantage of achieving quick results. Many hypnotherapists focus on teaching you methods, so you don't have to return to them for sessions regularly.

Another option is to find one of the many audios to help you lose weight. These can be played at your convenience, even if you cannot play them while riding or whatever you need to do.

Is it working?

This is the burning question that we all have. Trying this strategy is probably not going to hurt, and there is proof that some people are improving. At least, it can help you relax, which all of you can benefit from. Apart from this, something you concentrate on is right, even if it sounds suspiciously like what doctors and scientists call placebo.

Yet hypnosis or self-hypnosis, at least for some people, can do what it claims to do. However, you'd have to do it regularly for at least a few months to give it a fair chance. It could work more efficiently if you do. But even if you had seen results, continuing the sessions at least once a day for a while would be a good idea.

Many do not expect hypnosis to operate on itsown. The whole point is, of course, that it should make it easier for you to stick to your diet, fitness routine, and other goals. Your conscious mind will, however, support it by trying your best to remain focused.

Since the emphasis of hypnosis is on your subconscious, the specific techniques that work best for you still have to be identified. In other words, you can try to find a healthy diet that works with your body (not all foods work well for everybody).

The same applies to exercise. You should not try to hypnotize yourself to enjoy it if you have always hated going to the gym. Work with your social patterns and use yourself in a way that matches your desires and preferences.

The real aim of weight loss hypnosis is to encourage you to do what you have to do without using so much effort to lose weight. If your subconscious mind is more in tune with your conscious goals, there is less risk of deception by cheating on your diet or skipping your workout.

Hypnosis may sound strange or dangerous to lose weight, but it is only another way to use your mind in a way that promotes your goals. It may not be for all, but if the idea sounds enticing or at least exciting, you may want to look at several weight loss possibilities with hypnosis.

Hypnosis may be described as an alternative awareness-raising technique that helps people to be highly sensitive to the suggestions of a hypnotist.This routine was accepted for psychoanalysis to treat mental diseases by reviving the harmful events that occurred to them in the past (in particular in children) and providing suggestions to support them.

Hypnosis can cure phobias. It can be used to reduce stress or tension and can help you stay calm before and during a big test. You willenjoy hypnosis.

Hypnosis may control blood flow and the various autonomous functions that are generally not consciously controlled. The relaxing reaction of hypnosis also changes the neurohormonal systems that regulate many of the functions of the body.

Weight loss hypnosis will help you get through when all else has failed. Itwill support you to achieve the weight loss you desire. Hypnosis can be directed at the root of the problem and focus on replacing healthy choices with specific actions or behaviors.

Hypnosis can also be used to relieve the symptoms ofanxiety attacks. These include the inability to focus, indecision, extreme sensitivity, disharmony, sleep interruptions, excessive sweating, and persistent muscle tension.

Hypnosis can assist with coping mechanisms so that when stress-inducing situations occur, you can deal with them more appropriately. Itcan be used in many different ways. For example, itmay also be a tool for managing pain, often used for burn victims and pregnant women.

The accumulated therapeutic effect of hypnotic statements in the subconscious portion of the mind increases healthy self-worth. Hypnosis may cause a person to do anything contrary to his will or contradicts his values.A hypnotherapist has principles that only conforms to the accepted adjustment.

Not only can hypnosis allow you to accomplish your achievements, but it can help you stay motivated to achieve these objectives. After several "hypnosis therapy" sessions, you can find more desire to live and have more potential than ever expected.

Understanding how effective hypnosis is done does not require a degree of psychotherapy. It is a clear definition of coercion and persuasion and the ability to manipulate the environment.Not only does hypnosis induce people to try, but it also persuades them that there is no choice.

It's not just about planting an enticing seed–it's about steering them by smart tactics of mental control, strategic hypnosis, and NLP.Despite its clinical name, NLP is only capable of controlling interaction–not ruling but controlling it. Most of us practice some kind of mind control or NLP every day.

Sometimes it helps us to manipulate thoughts, particularly if we want something and realize that we can't do otherwise. Marriages are an NLP hotbed.Why? Because husbands and wivesoften have extensive knowledge and understanding of one another, so they also have a strong comprehension of the triggers of conflict.

Let us say that a husband wants a new $500 living room TV, but he knows that his wife will probably not be doing that unless it is a contract. At the store, he leads her first to the most expensive models – those that cost 1,000 or 2,000.

The husband then takes her to the cheapest sets as he looks at the heavy price tag, saying, "Look, these are much more affordable, are they not? She feels they got a deal, and they leave with the one he chose.The woman may not have clung to a point, but yet she has been the unwitting target of the hypnotic influence of the mind.

The human mind is not equipped with an operator manual, which means that it can be guided to any path we think fit, provided we know how to do this. The benefits of knowing hypnosis and the influence of a hypnotic suggestion are clear – they can help us improve our jobs, date a lovely woman, or buy new TV sets.

Used car salesmen use hypnosis every day. When you sense the feeling as a customer after being unwittingly drawn in by high-pressure sales tactics, you have definitely become a target of NLP.

The foundation of mind control starts by understanding what motivates and excites people by mastering the art of perception and communication. Once you understand the further motives, desires, and triggers of individuals, this knowledge can be integrated into your own method of hypnosis.You can make them feel comfortable and charmed by implicitly referring to things you know they think are important, and you can control the perceptions of reality once they are relaxed.

Contrary to popular belief, a person doesnot need to be gullible or naive in order to be fooled or hypnotized. Studies show that most people are vulnerable to mild hypnosis, and around 10% are hypnotic to an extreme depth.

There is no indication that certain functions or functionality are appropriate for NLP when you sit with someone; you can presume that they are open to covert hypnosis, whether it's your love interest, your boss, or your colleague.

Whether someone thinks they are vulnerable to hypnosis or not is not a concern when dealing with people who are not conscious that they are hypnotized.

Hypnosis is simply a state of increased awareness that leaves the human mind exposed to suggestive influence. It doesn't mean that you have to "catch people like chickens" or trick them.

It works for comedy hypnotics and hypnotherapists, but it does not do much for ordinary individuals. What does that do? The desire to get others on our side.

Remember: we are hypnotized and mesmerized every day. We are looking for ways to get people on our wavelength.

Knowing how to exploit the world starts with the understanding that human beings do not really know their reality. Truth is interpretation only.The ability to influence this interpretation is one of the many advantages of hypnosis.

Why Hypnosis Script Fail

A hypnosis script consists of a summary of various hypnosis processes. A well-developed script for hypnosis should be easily understood. The hypnosis script must explain with utmost care and clarification every move involved in hypnosis. A person who reads the hypnosis script can misinterpret facts. In comparison to other directions, this study method puts the complete burden of comprehension on the reader. A reader who attempts to gain control of the human mind can inevitably experience self-invited difficulties.

The hypnosis script – a step towards improved hypnosis scripts generally describes what a professional is going to do to a client. Expert hypnotizers usually write scripts based on their experience. It helps them develop their awareness and can be used as a material of reference. But it may be difficult for a beginner to learn hypnosis from a script alone.

The sensation and originality of true hypnosis cannot be conveyed by a hypnosis script. When a hypnotist first interacts with a client, he must gain the customer's attention and trust. The way the client sounds and modulates his voice cannot be said through a hypnosis script. A script for hypnosis can only describe the process. For a student of the hypnosis script, visualization of many aspects needed for hypnosis is abstracted.

A hypnotist must meet different personalities with different problems. The hypnotist needs a flexible approach to tackle each question. The rigidity of written words in the hypnosis script in actual circumstances will not be used.

CAN WEIGHT LOSS HYPNOSIS HELP PEOPLE LOSE WEIGHT?

For many people, losing weight is not the desireof everybody. Many people with a prolonged metabolism find it is incredibly challenging to lose weight, so they are lost before they even try to achieve it. On the other hand, other people are not fully committed to achieving their goals of losing weight. We are too lazy to do daily workouts and too hard to manage what we eat, making it almost impossible to lose weight. People who have a psychological problem are not allowed to achieve their goals. Plus, for people who have successfully incorporated self-hypnosis in their lives, hypnosis can make a difference.

Many people are not aware of weight loss hypnosis, and most of the findings showed promising potential in the area of safe management of weight. Online websites providing self-hypnosis services have multiple success stories about the hypnosis of weight loss, making it one of the most common physical supplements.

Hypnosis for weight loss is known as a way to add to a person's physical exercise and workout routine, according to the American Journal of Clinical Hypnosis (Volume 18, Number 1). Weight loss through hypnosis works by giving a person the desire to develop realistic aspirations to achieve his or her goals. By offering constant positive encouragement and thoughtful advice, so that a person who performs self-hypnosis to reduce weight can continue to lose weight. This is the secret to the excellent achievement of weight loss by many persons.

If a person who wants to achieve something is inspired, he will be much more eager to fulfill his own goals. Since the body can only do that which the mind thinks, training the mind will give those who try to lose weight a significant boost. Apart from that, a positive person regulates his behavior, making it easier to accomplish everything he aims for. Hypnosis to reduce weight provides a person with all the necessary encouragement and opportunity to achieve his or her goal of losing weight, and this is the advantage of hypnosis for people who seek to live healthily.

Who is using weight loss hypnosis, and what is the treatment like?

Many people wonder how hypnosis works for weight loss. You are intrigued by the whole thing and want to know a bit more about how hypnosis can help you with weight loss. Many visit a hypnotist who will make people do the stuff they could not do, and that is real. Yet they assume the hypnotist can transform them into robots that obey the hypnotist blindly. This isn't real, however. The main goal is to make a healthy person's habits regular and pursue them indiscriminately, as they become lifestyles.

This is a continuous process, and several sessions are scheduled. Each follow-up session focuses on responses. The right responses will be strengthened, and the wrong responses neutralized.

Does weight loss occur?

Apart from cure from disorders, try hypnosis to lose weight! How do you ask? By shaping your mind and re-programming the destructive habits that you have associated with eating and exercising. Hypnosis improvesyour food intake and exercise habits right to the source. It helps you restructure certain unhealthy behaviors that you have developed over the years, so to speak by, "installing" new patterns.

The definition is quite necessary. We are often bombarded by harmful diet and exercise habits from childhood to adulthood, and practically from every viewpoint – from the parents, the other children in school, to the tasty TV ads and billboards that cater to food!

Weight-loss hypnosis is easily one of the top three weight-loss strategies which include diet and exercise. Hypnosis makes the first two more effective.

See now how the three best strategies for weight loss fit together? If you can change your perspective on weight loss: how you eat, how you exercise, and how you use hypnosis, wouldn't it make more sense for you both to be more successful?

After at least three days of hypnosis sessions with a trained, licensed hypnotherapist, you can begin to see positive changes. The secret to success is to use a weight loss package (cd or otherwise) regularly for the first two weeks.

It helps to "mount" your new thoughts, acts, and behavior. Then, shortly afterward (and interestingly too!), you will find that your new behavior concretizes!

Would self-hypnosis work for weight loss? See if hypnosis will help you lose weight healthily!

The reality is that self-hypnosis has become a phenomenon in the field of weight loss. In a time when people are trying to get rid of the spare tire around their bellies, the unfortunate side effect is that some people get bamboozled. Not all programs are successful. You need to determine whether a hypnosis session online or in-person works better. In many areas of the country, there are also extensive group sessions.

Is hypnosis helping you to lose weight? The answer is yes, in some situations. Everything that the mind believes and sees is the truth. The reason specific self-hypnosis programs work is due to the right direction of the subconscious mind. Your brainwill find whatever you say to the subconscious mind.

Self-hypnosis can be used to lose weight, avoid cravings, enjoy nutritious foods, and learn to love exercise. Train your mind to believe that apples may seem more appealing than a bucket of chicken, for example. Nevertheless, a qualified hypnosis specialist will help you learn a new way to think about diet and exercise.

You must naturally equate every approach with healthy eating and exercise. The best way to create a roadmap for living a life with healthy habits is by using diet and exercise strategies. It is also usefulin keeping track of your diet. Hypnosis is only one of many forms of weight loss.

There are so many ways of losing weight and so many options to choose from. If you don't have time to invest in self-hypnosis, it's best to start the process of getting on track first with a plan.

MASTERING THE MAGIC OF HYPNOSIS: HYPNOTICS FOR WEIGHT LOSS.

After the discovery, the brain plays a vital role in weight loss. It plays a more significant role than most people think or imagine. People who were not on a weight loss program may not understand this easily.

The human fault is often said to be being overweight. You might also have learned that you must stop eating and start exercising to lose weight. Most people who struggle with weight management have taken part in a many programs to lose this weight, but with little or no positive results.

Although it is essential to identify factors that cause weight gain and may discover why the previous attempts to lose weight have failed, it does not go beyond this. Some people argue that obtaining knowledge and information about the cause of weight loss and why efforts to lose weight failed is part of the struggle.

If you know it's half the weight loss fight; you can call it the most natural part. Everyone who wants to lose weight already has some idea of what holds them back. What they don't know is how this situation can change.

Talk therapy has become very common these days in which people traintheir minds and regulate their body weight better. There are several forms of speech therapy, but weight loss hypnosis has become essential. Even if it sounds like an old concept, hypnosis is one of the recovery methods commonly used byhealth care professionals and weight loss clinics, as the effectiveness in most patients is high.

The weight loss hypnosis is preferred and is prescribed for fast results than long-term clinicaltherapy or psychoanalysis. Hypnosis is a unique approach because it focuses primarily on the positive aspects that have led to a change in the patient's mind and body.

While most psychoanalysis approaches seek to examine the causes of weight loss problems, hypnosis quickly moves through and removes these barriers and in addition to that, provides a rapid weight loss path. Hypnosis may simply be described as the ability to re-write your unconscious and conscious habits and thoughts.

Weight loss hypnosis uses encouragement and repetition. The sessions usually consist of 20 to 30 minutes of guided and repeated meditation every day. Once applied for an ongoing 30-day cycle, the brain adopts a new pattern or habit of thought.

In many instances, the human brain processes everything it experiences or sees through various levels of consciousness. Once a person first hears or sees something, it's stored in the short memory of the brain. The data that isstored in the short-term memory is repeatedly used as a permanent stamp on the mind, which leads to new habits or beliefs.

Self -hypnosis – Can you do it at home?

More and more people are now turning tohypnosis.So, why do you turn to weight loss self-hypnosis, is it because it works? Weight loss hypnosis works as well as hypnosis works for other anxiety or emotional issues that we humans have. We can go to hypnotherapists for almost every anxiety, phobias or mental problems, and they will help us with any issues for a heavy fee at times. So, where does self-hypnosis come in for weight loss?

The significant developments in the field of hypnotherapy, this is mainly due to the Internet, allows hypnosis for weight loss to be done thanks to CDs and DVDs with the use of new techniques manually created in audio format. The technologies enable people to purchase tailored self-hypnosis sessions for weight loss, for example, or a variety of subjects.

Many programs of top hypnotherapists are available online. So, you don't have to pay a hypnotherapist high rates anymore in light of the fact that they may not be all that good. You now have the opportunity to try your weight loss hypnosis in the comfort of your home using the software you can choose from amongst the many on the Internet. Please check credentials carefully when searching for a program and choose a program with which you are confident and, when buying a program, ensure it hasa money-back guarantee.

If you want to try self-hypnosis of weight loss, search the Internet wisely, and correctly test the reputation of the programmaker! Ok, not so good? Look for system testimonies, e.g., quality, successful use, or web support. You don't want to spend your hard-earned cash on a plan that's not right for you. Some women succeed with some programs quite well, and one of the best things with most programs is that they need little or no effort! Everything is from the comfort and security of your own home and you can afford it at a discount.

Weight Loss Hypnosis – A DIY Guide!

Let's make it simple. It is your brain that regulates what you do. The mind is responsible for the body. This is a simple concept, which we are all aware of. Nevertheless, when it comes to achieving goals, we can often be distracted by external factors, of which we have little or no influence. Those who want to lose weight often struggle due to genetics or bone structure, their hormones, or some other health factor about which we have no influence. It's just a diversion. In life, we must all work with what we now have, not how we want it to be. In reality, the'blame game' should be stopped altogether. It is most definitely unproductive, as well as exhausting and demotivating to blame ourselves, others, the universe, etc.

What is crucial is to understand that to achieve new goals, we have to change our thoughts, and only by improving our mindset can we change our actions.

I'm not only talking about changing what we say. Sure, this is important, but our unconscious thoughts are much more critical to change. The emotional/subconscious mind directly influences our behavior. All early psychiatrists and neurologists like Freud, Charcot, and Jung, recognized this reality.

Freud likened the mind to an iceberg that is as small as the conscious mind as the visible part, and that more in-depth, more significant, driving portion of our consciousness is hidden below the surface.Since it is the subconscious mind that drives actions and behavioral change are necessary for new purposes, how do we reach that part of the mind?

Self-hypnosis weight loss – how to make long-lasting changes to your lifestyle to help you lose weight

The use of self-hypnosis for weight loss is becoming increasingly popular in recent days. I agree that celebrities who use it to improve different aspects of their lives, so we should not be afraid of using that powerful tool.

Hypnosis is nothing mystical, and in its purest sense, you offer yourself or are given constructive feedback (by hypnosis) in a deeply relaxed state. The reality is that all of us are having every day hypnotic trances, but sadly most of us are working on pessimistic and ineffective suggestions.

Set aside a particular time of the day to monitor your thoughts and the pictures that you run in your mind. It will make beautiful things happen in your life.

Self-hypnosis for weight loss or any other purpose starts with learning how to relax, breathe properly, think, and affirm completely. The more we practice, the better we get, as with all we do in life. Your first hypnotic lesson is not as effective as the second and the second less effective than the third, etc. Using guided imagery such as beautiful scenery, sea waves, and a refreshing, friendly brisk breeze on the skin can help you completely relax and become highly suggestive. Then you imagine and validate your desired weight, food, and exercise.

Nearly every other day, I use hypnosis to strengthen different aspects of my life and must be honest here and state that improvements are not going to happen overnight. Currently, you need approximately a month of regular use to show results. Yet one thing I know for sure is that self-hypnosis works because of weight loss experienced.

USING SELF-HYPNOSIS – DOES IT WORKS?

Self-hypnosis can be a powerful tool to eliminate negative behaviors. This method has not only shown success with problems with weight loss and smoking, but alsoother issues.

When you visit a hypnotist, they will bring into your mind an idea, from which you can work when you need it most. Perhaps to lose weight, they'll tell you that if you want to eat fewercalories, you can eat vegetables.

It will depend on what you choose to do, but the rest of the process is very straightforward and simple. See, people enter a hypnotic process, and sometimes they don't even know it.

Have you ever driven home, and you do so without much thought? Every day you travel the same route. You are in a hypnotic trance at this stage, and your mind operates autonomously.

That is how you can use self-hypnosis for weight loss; if you start feeling hungry, you should go intothat trance. With the suggestion that has been made, the mind will do whatever it is told to do automatically.

Many people would think this is all a bunch of lies, but it has been studied to see how 90% of the population can be hypnotized. Perhaps this method is much more used and used for positive means. Consider trying to control hypnosis pressure and other issues in our lives that are difficult to get through.

A great way to at least try your weight loss is to visit a hypnotist to see if they can show you how to use the technique to drop the required pounds.

How you can make weight loss hypnosis a success

Many people are expected to lose weight by following the right diet and waiting for the weight to drop, and sometimes that's the case. Until everything comes back with a little extra, just days after the diet has ended. Given these interactions and those who don't see any pounds lost, people continue to move from one diet to the next. Not only is it deeply depressing to become involved in this yo-yo eating loop, but it can also cause more severe problems for health and mental well-being. The real secret to permanently losing weight lies in the psychological approach and the relationship to food. The recorded weight loss hypnotist knows this.

Thebest weight loss hypnosis is structured to use a combination of hypnotherapy and new language technology to soothe a patient's mental activity so that they can focus on the root problem. It is essential to understand that these therapies can only operate with the patient's full dedication before a course is taken. Unless that is the case, it will not be the desired success.

As the patient is gently stimulated, often to soothing music or gentle voice, theybecomes relaxed and comfortable. Completely aware of where they are and their surroundings, this allows the conversation to be centered entirely and explicitly. Hence, the therapist begins to discover why the negative relationship with food is established. Once these are determined, solutions can be sought and proposed to counter the thinking processes and memories causing the problem.

Once the therapist and patient have been taken out of induction, clarify the procedure to ensure everything is comfortable. A further "aware" debate follows on how ideas can best be applied in everyday life. Eventually, a discussion will take place in a controlled environment, and adjusted as appropriate to address other alternative therapies, such as exercises that will increase the effectiveness of hypnosis.

These techniques, which are carefully managed and adapted to individual requirements, would allow a more sustainable approach to food. The patient knows their underlying problems better, how to cope with them when they arise, and how to reduce the number of episodes. This is not a procedure intended to cure the problem, but to provide a way to help the patient recover.

So, does weight loss hypnosis succeed? The response should be yes, but only with lifestyle changes with commitment and awareness. Hypnosis will not give the weight a magical spell and keep it away, but it can allow patients to relax and to understand better how and why necessary changes work.

Do you think weight loss through hypnosis takes a long time? Think again. Find out how you can quickly slim down with the power of Begin Slim Hypnosis within five weeks or less

How do I get a great body by practicing weight loss hypnosis?

If you are under hypnosis, you are so relaxed that anyone (or even you) can recommend healthy, positive thoughts to your unconscious mind by self-hypnosis. This is the best way to explain any negative beliefs that hinder or kill oneself. This can, of course, only be done with your permission and active participation.

People usually hypnotize for weight loss using arguments. Tell yourself affirmations asrevolutionary goals you want to pursue. For instance, if you're going to will your weight from 200 to 150 pounds, you probably say, "Now I weigh 150 pounds," or "Easily I lose 50 pounds," often; hypnosis is used to encourage people to live up to their expectations or to maintain discipline. For example, if you have difficulty keeping your diet to lose weight and exercise to gain muscle weight, you can recommend thoughts in your subconscious mind such as why you can keep your diet, how to get your perfect body shape, work out programs, and safety advantages.

In this way, you program your subconscious mind to lose weight or practice to minimize expectations and develop more positive thoughts and beliefs that will help you adhere to your diet. That is why I suggest which weight loss hypnosis is an excellent alternative to reducing the body's excess fat.

HYPNOSIS OF WEIGHT LOSS – NO MORE HYPNOTIZATION

Not many people try hypnotic weight loss. The main reason is that until now, hypnosis is related to illusions and frustration rather than a legitimate treatment option. However, many cultures around the world have practiced this ancient art for millennia to treat several physical and mental disorders, including addictions, sleeping problems, depression, etc. Thousands of people have embraced weight loss hypnosis as one of the most workable, non-invasive treatment options for successful weight loss.

To believe that hypnosis can help to lose weight, you first have to assume that gaining weight has more to do with the body than with the mind. If you accept this basic fact, you will also believe in a loss of weight using hypnosis. The mode of action of hypnotherapy is to enter the depths of your subconscious, where most of our worries and inhibitions lie and address the root of the problem of obesity. Any medicine or diet program will touch the mind, of course.

To understand how hypnosis helps to lose weight, you have to realize that all the anxiety, phobia, emotions, and thoughts have their origins at the subconscious level of the mind. This stage is usually dormant, except when we dream. Surprisingly enough, this subconscious level determines how we act and how we shape habits. For example, we make many poor lifestyle choices, become addicted to the wrong drugs, and eat the wrong kinds of food–all rooted in subconsciousness.

The hypnosis process begins with relaxation techniques that relax the mind. This relaxed state is necessary to be responsive to constructive feedback and affirmations inserted externally at the subconscious level. This stage will awaken from the sleeping state and also become confessional. Hypnosis creates a restored link between the conscious and the unconscious mind in other dimensions.

There are several reasons for an overweight person to lose weight, among them the need for energy, money, love, and attention. Hypnosis tackles all these issues and resolves them through more constructive and logical auto recommendations. It frees the mind from all negative aspects and gives it a new direction. You are soon to make the right choices in your life because hypnosis for weight loss has changed your thinking. The best thing about this therapy choice is for you to build a new approach to weight loss.

Many people wonder how hypnosis works for weight loss. Maybe theyare intrigued by the entire process and want to know a bit more about how hypnosis can help them with weight loss.

Most people visit a hypnotist who believed hypnosis would allow them to do something they could not, and that is real. But they think the hypnotist can make them robots in which they only blindly follow the hypnotist. This isn't real, however. The main goal is to make a healthy person's habits normal and to adopt them "blindly" because they have become habits.

After hypnosis, it's much easier to practice healthy habits because your mind is used to new behaviors.

You can now officially practice hypnosis with the aid of a trained hypnotherapist or use it yourself. Several dimensions of hypnosis should be achieved:

1. Relaxation. This makes it possible to relieve the' essential facility' of the prefrontal cortex. Slowing down the necessary facility ensures that improvements in the deeper regions of the mind are more likely to be accepted.

2. Visualization/emotional alert. Good-fitting emotions or visualizations linked to emotional states help us to influence the mental "subconscious" mind directly.

3. A suggestion that is hypnotic. A second party will make the best suggestions, including hypnotic suggestions for weight loss. Suggestions made by someone else seem to be more successful than the suggestions given to you. But it's also powerful to make suggestions to yourself you can genuinely believe in.

It doesn't matter whether it's hypnosis for weight loss, depression hypnosis, success, or motivation. Follow thesesimple steps:

1. Relax in a comfortable spot. Youcan either sit or lie down. Then close your eyes.

2. Start with your feet, slowly clamp and relax each muscle group in your body until you hit the top of your head. Concentrate on each muscle group as far as you can. Note the muscles in your abdomen in particular.

3. Once you relax your abdomen's muscles, take three slow deep breaths to make sure your abdomen grows. Don't breathe in the chest. This is the time to let it hang out.

4. Breathe normally and start relaxing. Rememberholding and rubbing the back, spine, upper arms, lower arms, and hands.

5. Try to relax the face and jaw muscles, if possible, by first clamping them.

6. Check your body mentally and relax with any places you like.

7. Introduce mental stimulation by imagining disturbing thoughts or nagging feelings. You may want to believe them floating away or vanishing into a brume or breathing out with every breath.

8. Visualize a favorite venue. This can be a place from your memory or a place in your imagination. You will feel relaxed and secure somewhere. Take time to imagine every item that exists in this place – the floor, the walls, the view, and so on. Always imagine the feeling of being there.

9. Remember the old feeling from which you want to switch. It might be a feeling of craving junk food or a sense of disappointment with a small meal or a feeling of fear that exceeds

the secondary sensations. Think what the feeling is that drives your behavior; then note it. Feel it if you can for a few moments and now turn to a substitute feeling as soon as possible. The alternative feeling is one of happiness, fullness, relaxation, accomplishment, or achievement. Call on a pleasant memory or imagined scenario to create a new emotion. Do this at least three times.

10. Recall any powerless'former' feelings. Replace them with a new thought that is more beneficial. For example, replace: "One more is ok" by "I have the right to choose what I put in my body" or "I choose to control myself." Tell yourself the new thoughts, and understand the new feelings associated with this modern, more balanced approach as much as possible. You might imagine erasing the old ideas by wiping them off a chalkboard. Do this at least three times with every helpless thought you have found.

11. Anchoring the fresh feelings and thoughts by bringing the thumb and forefinger together. Instead, relaxation in a different part of your body could be taken into consideration. You could also recall a music piece or say a sentence in your mind that reminds you of this state.

12. Remember the old conduct. Only picture it as much as you can, as it was a TV scene or film screen. Just imagine you had a click for rewinding. Press rewind to return to the beginning of the sequence, then play events again, with the new behavior. Again, do it at least three times.

13. Talk to yourself,' This old problem is diminishing, and every day I step away from old conduct and old faithfulness: 'I build a new destiny.'

14. When you are ready, gently return to a healthy state of consciousness and open your eyes.

The entire process should take approximately 10 to 30 minutes.

When you do this, use your anchor (the thumb and forefinger touch or stimulation in the part of your body or phrase) many times when you need to feel and remember the manner you want to do it. Make sure that your thoughts and emotions are sufficient to overcome the problem. If not, you will need to practice more often or seek professional assistance.

I encourage you to do this onetime a week and then once or twice a week until you are sure that new ideas, emotions, and actions will be firmly established.It's easy to change your emotions, feelings, and actions by hypnosis once you practice it sometimes.

Best wishes to meet your full potential!

WHAT YOU MUST FOCUS ON TO LOSE WEIGHT (IT'S NOT THE POUNDS)

A pound of fat includes about 3500 calories. You have to use 3500 more calories than you consume to lose a pound of fat; although it seems like a straightforward explanation, note that your body is a thought-protecting organism.

If one day you tried to reduce your intake by 3500 calories, your body will record some kind of warning and assume there is a state of emergency. Your metabolism would slow down immediately, and there would be no weight loss.

You will spread your weight loss over one week to reduce your caloric intake by 3500 to 7000 calories per week, resulting in a weekly weight loss of 1 to 2 pounds. It is not usually advisable to try to lose over 2pounds a week. Attempting to do so can lead to health risks.

For starters, you can use a simple calorie-counting method to help you achieve your target by trying to lose two pounds per week. For this reason, you need to find out how much calories you usually need in a day for a person of your age, sex, and weight, take 500 from that number and follow a diet that offers you that many nutrients.

For example, if you typically need 3,000 calories a day, you should follow a daily diet of 2500 calories. Figure out how much a person of your weight needs to exercise to burn 500 calories a day and choosea workout plan that will help you achieve your objective.

The effect is simple: 500 fewer calories and 500 additional calories not consumed equal to a 1000 calories daily deficit, which corresponds to up to 7,000 or 2pounds over a week. Even if the results vary, if your body absorbs fewer calories than it uses, then the weight will be lost.

Here are eight tips to help you quickly lose weight

1. Please read food labels: attention should be paid to food labels, and the calorie content and serving size should be known. You tend to make healthier choices as you learn to compare food labels.

2. Intelligent snacking: It might seem paradoxical to tell you that eating small portions can help you lose more weight, but it works. Seek to get safe and adequate snacks such as an apple and a fatty cheddar cheese to avoid becoming too hungry at the next meal.

3. Say yes to grains and produce: whole grains, fruit, and vegetables contain fiber that keeps you full long-term. These are also low in calories, which means you are less likely to eat other unhealthy foods.

4. Stop skipping meals: skipping meals is not a way to lose weight. On the other hand, this makes you binge at the next meal, and also the body is hungry, making you gain weight!

5. Water, water and more water: more water helps you stay away from sodas and fruit drinks which are full of calories. Water also relieves fluttering and enhances the overall well-being feeling. Thirst can affect your appetite, and if you drink less water, you will consume more.

6. Get moving: no way can you lose weight or stay fit without exercise. Also, simple exercises like walking for 20 minutes a day are more than necessary. Exercise has many other health benefits and also improves metabolism.

7. Portion control: measuring the size of food portions can seem tedious, but the attempts to lose weight are invaluable. However, when you know how to calculate servings, you might realize that you had tocorrect the serving size two or three times before beginning a weight loss program.

8. Put it down in writing: you first need a food diary if you want to lose weight. Write down what, when, and how much you eat so that you can have an idea of improving your current eating habits. Yeah, this diary can even be done online on one of StripThatFat's best weight loss programs.

Established strategies to prevent overweight

If you've ever tried to lose weight, you know how difficult it is to prevent obesity. Once you are ona diet, how often do you look for reasons to say, it's okay, have a cake or a pizza slice? If you're like me, quite often. The problem is that once I've had "forbidden food,"

I tell myself that I might go and eat that I want to have the rest of the day and get fresh tomorrow. Tomorrow, I tell myself, on Monday, I'm going to wait and get a new beginning. You know what I'm talking about if you are a career dietitian.

There are several cases in which I repeat this loop over and over.I'm going to share four of these scenarios and what I do to solve the issue.

Place #1–Christmas parties and social events, birthdays, anniversaries, weddings, etc. What they all share in common is an abundance of food. When you're offered a piece of cake or cheese dip, other guests will encourage you to try a little. They tell you the one piece won't hurt; it's a special occasion. Soon then you've taken a nibble and eat more and more. You're bloated and embarrassed before you know it.

How do I stop it: I will enjoy a big healthy meal just before I leave, so I'll be full for a couple of hours. If I am hungry like I usually am, the veggie tray is the first thing I'll go for. Many vegetables are not available so that a small amount of food information comes in handy. Find other healthy alternatives on the list. If there are full grain bread sandwiches, you are in good shape. If not, throw away the bread and enjoy a ham or turkey slice. Just stay away from the wings and chips. When you are asked to bring a plate, make sure that you have a healthy snack. I carrieda veggie tray or flavored rice cakes several times. Choose the best food and eat a small portion if you have no choice.

Situation #2 — Partner or other serious sabotage. It is challenging to eat healthy when your partner or other important person does not actually consume the same food. They don't try to sabotage your diet; they just don't want to make good food choices.

How do I stop it: my wife doesn't always eat the same stuff I do, but it's all right. We usually make enough chicken or fish for a few days. So, I still have a good lunch, snack, or dinner option. I boil broccoli, heat a piece of chicken, and we are both satisfied when my wife decides she wants garlic pasta. I will choosethe healthiest option on the menu and eat sensibly when she insists on Chinese food. I just make sure that it's the exception, not the law.

Situation #3–You don't see yourself as overweight when you look at the mirror.

How do I avoid it? I sometimes look into the mirror and say, "You don't look overweight." When I see a picture, my response changes, it's more like,'Oh, my gosh, I can't believe how fat I look.' Take your worst fat image and keep it with you. Every time you decide you want a pizza slice, view the photo.

Situation #4— all or nothing mentality; that's my worst enemy.

How I prevent it.That's the worst thing for me. I also find that I can't just stop it, so we compromise. We usually decide that I'm too weak. She respects and supports my health efforts. Instead, we will choose to make our pizza. How good a whole grain tortilla, grilled chicken, fat-free, tomato sauce, ointment, and turkey bacon-flavored be! Would you be shocked! Occasionally she orders a pizza, but she gets a personal size or the next one. So, if I slip into temptation, it won't be too much to feed me.

You've always been looking for tips that might help you lose weight. Such tips are useful for you. You realize that some weight loss tips may work for you, while others cannot work for you.

Right here, you can read some ideas you can pursue weight loss. These are, of course, not expected to help you completely lose all your excess weight. You understand that every person is unique and so a tip that can work for you, and vice versa. You have to decide whether you want to try a weight loss tip. It can lead you to weight loss. However, if it doesn't, don't say all other weight loss ideas are myths, because some of them work for you.

One of the most popular ways of losing weight is to workout or do a physical job. The probability of consuming the calories you take is quite high if you are very healthy and have an active lifestyle. You're going to have a slimmer body than others. The more exercise you do, the more calories you consume. It ensures that your body can store fewer calories. You know the additional calories are converted into fat.

You can try to do something else if you can't do physical activities. Instead, you should guarantee that your consumption is just 500 fewer calories throughout the day. Therefore, you can be sure that your body will burn it well. It's not too much to take from your body.

You can also note how many calories you eat every day. You could limit your intake in this way. It is said that if you take note of every bite of food you consume, you will know what you eat. If that happens, you will realize how much you eat, and unconsciously, you will decrease that amount.

You must choose what you eat. It is essential. Your body needs fat, but you're still on the good side if you want the right kind of fat. You can use virgin olive oil rather than butter. You can haveall milks. You can also go fishing for fat. Both olive oil and fish fat are right for your heart.

How many days do you eat? How many hours? You may not be on the road to weight loss if you consume three meals each day. What you can do instead is eat often in small quantities. It will help you lose the extra pounds. Those who tried to do this will tell you it works.

FIVE PERMANENT WAYS TO ACHIEVE CONSTANT WEIGHT LOSS!

I feel your pain. Few things are as frustrating as putting sweat and pain to lose that awful weight just to fall off the wagonand to see that weight come back with a vengeance. Don't worry, please. Let's concentrate instead on five easy ways to achieve a successful weight loss!

Diets don't work!

If you love to eat, it's the best news you've ever seen. Diets don't work! Many people confuse what a diet is for which certain bodyweight is to be reached by a specific date. Of course, when you are an athlete or fitness model, diets are needed to achieve a bodyweight by a specific date, but the diet is doomed to failure in terms of making a lasting weight loss.

What a diet does is limit the amount of food you can consume and what food you can eat. Dieting is very painful. When you take your favorite food away, it will only be a matter of time before you are tempted.

Adjust Lifestyle!

The people who succeed in getting the weight off and keeping it off were those who changed their way of life! They decided to change their daily habits (that used to be overweight and shapeless. They heard about proper nutrition and exercised daily in their way of life.

They have changed the image of themselves from couch potato to committed health care workers who have taken care of their health and well-being!

Daily preparation! Regular practice!

To finally achieve permanent weight loss, you just need to exercise daily. This is part of the change in lifestyle that I mentioned just now. Regular exercise contributes to accelerating the metabolism that leads to fuel burning. The trick is to find a kind of exercise that you like or at least don't hate. So you can stay with it long enough to see results!

Eat more often!

What?! That's right. One of the secret tricks to lose weight is to eat more often. Instead of typical three meals a day, seek six smaller meals throughout the day. When eating more often, you reduce the risk of hunger, which contributes to eating. Obviously, for your six smaller meals, you want to choose healthier food choices.

The Veggies Load Up!

Here is some excellent news in the fat fight. Seek every meal with plenty of raw or lightly steamed vegetables. Not only are vegetables rich in nutrients and low in calories, but because of their high fiber content, they are also very satisfying. This means you can have nearly unlimited quantities of vegetables with no weight gain. Adding vegetables to your diet will satisfy you after eating.

You can achieve a significant loss of weight by recognizing that diets do not work for long term weight management. A change in lifestyle, regular exercise, and loading on vegetables do though. Is it going to be easy? No, but a little effortis simple; otherwise, we would all live our dream lives. These five simple changes will lead you to a slimmer, more pleasant life.

Weight loss cleansing or weight loss detox products

Your thinking is one of the most important aspects of weight management. With the wrong way of thinking, you defeat yourself before you begin. You can produce spectacular results much faster than you can imagine with the right mindset.

If you're like most of us, you're not one of the 1 million of us struggle to lose weight only to rebound once the diet is over. If so, you most likely use the internet to look for new and different weight loss products. When most of us think about the loss of weight, diet pills are usually the first thought. While diet pills can be a good product to help you achieve your goals for weight loss, diet pills are not good for everyone. Many people have found a free and easy weight loss method using colon cleansing to lose weight quickly and effectively. Such products are usually referred to as weight loss cleansing or weight loss detox products and allow you to achieve free, easy weight loss. These are little-known products, which make losing 10 pounds very easy.

When it comes to using colon cleansing to reduce weight, many people are surprised, maybe just like you, about the way the method works. It's important to remember, before learning how they can help you achieve free,natural weight loss, that there are numerous cleanses. Some of them are primarily designed to help you lose weight. These are usually called cleanses for weight loss, and it is designed for detoxifying the body. But ultimately, they both work in the same way.

You must follow all the instructions given to you when using any kind of cleansing product. For example, some products claim you should eat nothing for one or two days. Usually, these varieties are in liquid form. Those who come in pill form may mean that you just eat and drink those things, such as fruit and vegetables. If there is a product which recommends that you restrict your diet, it is advisable to try. This dietary restriction helps you to lose weight and allow the drug to work properly.

You can detoxify your body with a colon cleansing drug. It functions to protect the colon and intestines from poisons. Not only will this cycle clean up your system, but it will also help you lose weight. It is said that the average person has poisonous rotting food in their bodies from four to eight pounds. This extra waste is removed from your body when using a colon cleanse. This is only one reason you lose weight.

ARE YOU TRYING TO LOSE WEIGHT?

Thousands of people all around the world are willing to do anything to decrease their weight. The easiest way to lose weight is to reduce your food intake and stick to a healthy diet. It is also good to drink plenty of water because it is an effective way to lose abdominal fat.

Some tips for weight loss

The first and most important recommendations are to look at what you eat and to drink more water. All you need to do is keep the balance correct and count every slice. You must know how many calories your body requires and then prepare your diet accordingly.

Another essential thing to bear in mind is that diets don't work during weight loss. If you follow some diet plan, in a few months, you will recover all the weight loss because diets are temporary. You must improve your dietary lifestyle so that you can continue to succeed. Avoid crash diets as they are dangerous rather than healthy.

If you try to lose weight, joining a support group will be a great help. Many online support groups are available, and you can also build your own. It is easy to be overwhelmed, depressed, alone, and lose hope. It's a wise move to meet friends or relatives. You will often be aware that you are not the only one struggling, and many people will share their wisdom and secrets with you. You will share with them tears, laughter, stories, mistakes, and achievements.

It is also a good idea to take pictures only for records before and after. Sharing your images with others will be fun, and they could calculate whether you improved. Make sure you eat five portions of fruit and vegetables each day when you are filled with beneficial vitamins, fibers, and antioxidants for your weight loss. They make you feel full and they are low in calories, too.

You need to look at the portion size to maximize it. You need to know the portion, as one portion of the pasta is half a cup of cooked pasta. When you eat out, the portion is usually much smaller, but note that you don't have to finish everything and ask to take the leftovers home.

One of the most ignored suggestions is to avoid eating. You need to eat small traditional meals, so your calorie intake is balanced all day long. Eating 5-6 smaller meals also maintains a healthy blood sugar level.

Try to buy fresh food items rather than processed and fast foodones during weight loss, as they are high in fat and sodium content. Pack your home-cooked lunch instead of dining out when you work.

An essential aspect of such a system is the awareness of food labels. A fat-free product does not mean fewer calories. Therefore, low fat or low sugar does not mean low calories or fat. Try to read the nutrition label correctly and understand it well.

Most people have realized that it can be beneficial to keep a food journal during weight loss. It allows you to recognize and change your eating patterns. You can also ask your registered dietitian to review your food journal once in a while to make sure you choose the right foods.

Most experts recommend that you remain fit and healthy by exercising for at least 30 to 60 minutes every day. You can also try adding weight-training exercise two to three days a week because that helps to burn extra calories.

Whatever form of weight loss you select, ensure the weight loss is progressive. Learn to make healthy food choices and take advantage of your workout.

Quick And Easy Weight Loss Tips

The quest for shortcuts and quick performance is only part of human nature. The problem is that if you lose weight too soon, you'll be right back to square one. Here are some tips for weight loss that will motivate you to reach successful weight loss and look forward to a lifetime of healthiness.

Weight loss tip #1: maintain a one-week food and exercise log. Keep track of daily calories and calories burned daily. Don't lie! Don't cheat! Put it all down. It is a critical step towards weight loss, to be honest with you. At the end of the week, you'll have a good idea about your average daily calories. Then go to the next weight loss tip and decide what you should eat per day.

Weight loss tip #2: learn the basic weight loss formula. Calories must be equal to calories. We all have a certain amount of calories that our current weight needs: our level of height, weight, sex, age, and exercise. Such calories are spent on the daily needs for our physical activities, such as respiration and digestion, and our usual duties, whatever they may be. Use a calorie calculator to calculate this amount of calories. If you want to lose weight, two things must be done:

1. Lower this intake of calories.

2. Increase the amount of burned calories.

Weight loss tip #3: with time, there will be a safe, sustainable weight loss. One to two pounds a week is the guideline. A pound of fat is equivalent to approximately 3500 calories. Therefore, you need a calorie deficit of 500 calories a day if your target is to lose one pound a week. If you want two pounds a week, the deficit should be 1000 calories per day. If you have decided that your calories per day are 2000 calories, then reduce your consumption to 1750 per day and consume another 250 calories per day. It could be so easy as a half sandwich for lunch and a brisk two-mile walk instead of a whole sandwich. If you want to reach a weight loss of two pounds per week, don't raise your calories too dramatically.

Tip for weight loss #4: read food labels. Nobody wants to spend all their days counting the calories they put in their mouths. At first, knowing portion sizes and caloric amounts areessential, but you will be able to ballpark most of what you consume after some time. You'll probably also be shocked at the outset. It doesn't seem fair that half a cup is a servingof ice cream! As hard as it is, you have to learn so that you realize that filling the cereal bowl with what you once used eat is more than 1000 calories when you think you eat 350 calories of unreduced fat ice cream. One sliceof bread is a serving ng size, typically about 100 calories. I began eating sandwiches open-faced when I found out this.

Weight loss tip #5: be mindful that what you are doing now is one of the main things you can do for yourself! Functional, permanent loss of weight is an unbeatable reward for all your hard work. The secret is patience. Don't pay attention tothe co-worker who lost 10pounds to any fad diet she attempted last week! I guarantee you in five to six weeks, she will have gained back much of it, and you will reap the rewards of your easy, steady weight loss; not only that but the skills and expertise you will have built up to keep the weight away for good!

IS EXERCISE GOOD FOR YOU AND YOUR DIET?

What is the truth, and how much risk is exercising on a diet is for you?

Activity

The majority of medical experts agree that the healthy human body is designed for a life that involves physical activity. The negative health consequences of not doing enough exercise are now generally accepted. The resulting issues are established and can be a severe and life-threatening concern in places like the cardiovascular system.

From a nutritional point of view, exercise is essential as it takes lowers calories and reduces our body's food energy as fat.Therefore, from a variety of different perspectives, exercise is essential.However, the cumulative effects of this sedentary lifestyle have to be taken into account.

If you've been living a relatively inactive life for several years, there's a good chance your body may not be in the best physical shape now. Even if you are not overweight as such, take this into account before doing anything else than relatively modest physical exercise.

This is because subjecting an ineffective body to a very challenging and physically exhausting series of exercises can lead to potential medical problems.

Here's another question.Many people who have lived a relatively inactive lifestyle for a period may also have experienced a significant increase in weight. The possible medical risks of excessive exercise may even be increased if you are both unhealthy and overweight.If someone who is unhealthy and overweight faces risks when it comes to challenging work, should this be avoided totally?

The answer to the question above must be an emphatic no.

The human body is an extraordinary entity, and to a certain degree, is perfectly capable of fixing some of the harm caused by negligence in the fields of exercise and dietary practice over the years. Some conventional diet programs include some workout elements in their strategies, and the success stories are primarily around weight loss.

However, it can be unwise and risky to immediately follow a rigorous exercise regime without any knowledge of your physical capacities.

What is crucial is that you continue your workout according to your professional advice. This recommendation takes the age, weight, blood test indicators, and overall health into account. As a result, recommendations can be made on activities that are proportionate to your health and physical condition, and that represents a reasonable degree of risk.

Professional and medical guidance on all activities that are likely to be considered punitive or physically demanding in any way is always recommended.

Don't be hindered by the false belief that your doctor or dietician is surprised by your current condition or weight. You will have seen everything before and prescribe an effective exercise regime that takes particular circumstances into account.

We live in a world where everything is in a community where everything is exchanged. If you're too late, you're left behind, and no one wants to be left behind. They want to be at the pace in which the world moves. Whether it is the internet connection or perhaps how people rush about stuff doesn't matter. Everything is moving quickly. That even means you want to lose weight that way too. Many people want to know how to lose weight quickly. You don't know that it isn't just part of the fast-paced world because it takes time.

You cannot lose weight in just one or two days,. Now, if you want it so bad, you may need to diet at least a week or two. You should try the chickendiet. This is very common for those who want to lose weight quickly. So what's the cold diet? Okay, this one is about soup. The soup consists mainly of rice. It also includes other vegetables.

So, how's it going to work? See, you can eat a lot of soup with the chicken diet. Only on the first day should this happen. You should add other forms of healthy food to your diet the following days. You will realize, of course, that if you want a long-term diet to which you will follow, thisis not one. It's not so safe.

You should try the slim fast diet if you are looking for a short-term way to lose weight very quickly. This is usually announced by celebrities and people in the sports world on television. You'd have this program in diet shakes. These shakes will make you feel full and have fewer calories than if you'd eat a meal. It works for that purpose. But you shouldn't stick to it if you want to lose these pounds consistently for a long time. You don't have enough nutrients and vitamins in your body because you no longer eat correctly.

Now, if you want to lose weight quickly and healthily, consider the one effective way—exercise!

Exercise is very popularand is understood by nearly everybody. However, not many people like it. The trick to fitness, though, is to find the physical activity you like so much swimming or dancing, that you don't feel like exercising.

These are some of the suggestions you might consider if you want to learn how to lose weight quickly. We have their benefits and disadvantages, and it is up to you to see whatworks for you and who doesn't.

The quick weight-loss guide is the perfect weight

This provides simple health tips and nutritional tips to keep your body safe and balanced. A controlled diet can be beneficial in keeping the body fit. You can find easy tips on diet control and also find tips on your weight loss diet plan, which are easy to follow and are therefore useful in preserving your health.

It is not all about a balanced and sustained diet to preserve your health; regular exercise is also required to burn the additional calories that are consumed during the day. The guide provides easy and basic workouts, which are presented in a perfect way and are easy to understand for users so that it can be followed to keep the body healthy and fit.

A lot of fitness magazines and exercise books are also available that you can follow to keep your body fit. According to a simple guide to weight loss, the easiest way to be fit is to reduce calorie intake and increase calorie burning. The website also includes some videos and images for the activities you can see and perform. You don't have to go to the gym every day and practice there consistently, a simple guide to weight loss shows you the steps you can use in your everyday busy life and thus maintain a healthy environment by losing additional weight.

Experts recommend all recommendations, tips, and activities and seminars included in this study. Nutritionists, healthcare professionals, and weight loss experts provide health tips, so you don't have to worry about it before you comply.

There are many blogs and posts that offer regular and valuable health tips. Such fitness tips and exercises also help you increase your willingness and ability. If you follow the health tips provided by the weight loss easy guide, you can assess your health regularly. The weight loss tips here are helpful and can help you maintain your good health.

You may have to combat what the medications are meant to do for you. Recently, nutritional drugs and food supplements have been revealed to help you reduce weight.

The only downside for the vast majority of people is that the process is easy to use.

Disadvantages

- Can be relatively expensive.
- There is little knowledge of the long-term side effects of relatively new medications and food supplements.
- It does not deal with the root cause of weight gain, and thus, weight gain is almost unavoidable if supply is cut off.
- It can require a maintenance dose to keep weight stable.
- Low self-esteem can be shown in many, even less appropriate ways that can lead to additional treatment and a possible increase in weight.

It is relatively common for a drug to go through the clinical trials successfully and to be on the market for several years before unexpected removal because harmful long-term side-effects have been discovered.

Special diets such as a single diet, high protein diets, blood type diets, etc. are often the brainchild for people who are highly motivated to minimize their weight.

Advantages–

Use a prescribed diet, often in a book or other written format.

Certain procedures can help to eliminate frequent coughs, and cold drawbacks-It can be quite inflexible, costly, or both. Some of these diets are unhealthy, as well as liposuction and tummy tucks. Operating surgery takes three types. These are quite extreme ways of weight reduction and should be avoided if possible. Like all procedures in which large amounts of anesthesia are used, there is a risk of death.

Note, the surgeon and the clinic are investigating before you agree.

Advantages of liposuction-

- A potential radical transformation of the form of body and limb/size
- No effort required
- It can result in a long-term improvement if the character of a person is correct.
- Can be painful
- outcomes may be informative
- Special care requires for some days afterward. The outcome varies depending on the procedure of the surgeon, the skill, and the experience.

Losing Fat: The Fast And Simple Way

Losing fat is like riding a bicycle: you could fall over a couple of times, but when you hold on, you won't forget.

There are so many accounts of losing the fat everywhere in your body: your head, your back, your neck, your cheeks, everywhere! People would recommend that you do some exercises to' hit' the fat around this region. This could be the greatest amount of hogwash I've ever heard, and you understand why, once you are aware of the mechanics behind you losing fat!

How can we lose all this fat?

To understand how you lost it, consider first how you got it: lack of exercise–people see this as the number one reason that others are overweight. Although it has a lot of issues in the discussion, people still exercise, but don't lose weight! However, it has to be said that any exercise is better than no exercise every time.

Ask yourself honestly: have you eaten too much and too often those types of food? I am not here to warn you about consuming' clean and healthy' foods (a word that doesn't hold water is the idea people have of so-called' good' foods) all I want to do is to make you aware that your diet is the most crucial factor for your loss of weight.

Your biology can be blamed all day long, but genetics will not keep you from losing fat or push you to pick up that extra slice. Stop being a slave to this excuse and be responsible from here on for the decisions you make about your body.

It is now essential to consider these things to lose the fat mass that you have gained in your body: Setting goals–don't look at me like that. Writing your priorities on paper makes you always stick to the mission that you have set out to do. Think of how you are going to feel how your friends and family are going to react! You must want it before you can work towards it.

Diet: go to every section of the search engine and look for the "macro-nutrient calculator." You enter information including age, height, and current weight and measure how much you will eat per day to maintain your current weight, to lose weight or to gain weight. Now you will need to start tracking your food intake once you have the number (weight loss energy level). Without a map, you can't travel through a foreign country and expect to come to the right location.There are many applications for monitoring the consumption and breakdown of macro-nutrients.

Keep the fat intake low–while fats have a place in your diet, fat intake affects fat loss only because they are higher in energy than protein or carbohydrate and can easily exceed your energy goals.

Reduce sodium intake – 3 g of sodium is plentiful per day. You don't have to cut it off completely, just make sure you stay within this range. Excess sodium allows you to retain water weight and make your limbs look bigger.

Training–This may be clear to you, but you need to get up and do some kind of exercise! Run, jog, swim, walk— all you can think of!

Anything to increase the rate of your heart for at least 30 minutes every day or every otherday.

Eating more protein–Consuming protein has a thermogenic effect on your body, in which the protein source is metabolized and, in turn, increases the body's temperature to promote fat loss.

Drink more water – Water is what your body needs in all metabolic processes, like lipolysis.

Take cold showers–Getting into a cold shower might be the last thing to do after one long day, but it works to lose fat! The fall in body temperature is quite fast, and when you get out, your body will invest energy in a process called thermoregulation, which will lift your body temperature back to normal. Fat loss takes place because of the energy consumption the body requires to return the temperature to normal.

Eat more vegetables–Vegetables are packed with vitamins and minerals your body needs to act properly. They are also a high fiber source that helps clean the intestine and keep you healthy.

Say NO to sugar – Sugar is a very easy carbohydrate to digest. This generates sufficient energy to be used immediately. What do you think happens if you don't use the available energy? Yeah, it is stored as fat. Choose to digest slower carbohydrates, including brown rice, brown bread, oats, and sweet potato, to name a few. These will satisfyyou longer, lessen the cravings, and keep insulin spikes at bay if you consume them alone (with no protein or fat).

Live a balanced life– It's good to have a coke or spoil yourself with a chocolate bar once in a while. After all, we are people, so don't blame yourself for that. Make it part of your diet; leave room for yourself to be spoiled. All in moderation is by far the best way to live in harmony.

The path to a fantastic body is only driven by your readiness to change. You're incontrol, and it's time to understand that!

Tips for helping you lose weight

Many people look at themselves in a mirror and wonder how theylet go of their waistline. They then decide each day to make the necessary changes to help them continue losing the extra pounds. However, many people find it hard to control themselves or just do not have a clear understandingof tips on weight loss. If you have been searching for some helpful ideas that can help you reduce your weight, this text might help.

One of the many significant points for people trying to get rid of extra weight is that they have difficulty disciplining themselves. Sometimes, long hours and a hectic working life leave them feeling exhausted and unable to collect energy to eat properly or to function well.

Weight loss meetings are very useful for many individuals. While some people regularly meet with friends to discuss their issues and ambitions at local recreationcenters, others start their teams or enter online groups. You may even launch a group effort with a pal near you. Individuals who have helped tend to try and build and adopt a healthier lifestyle more easily.

The benefit of someone helping you is that they can come and help with your meals. You can also cook wholesome dinner foods to some degree. You can even agree to exercise together daily. At the end of every day or week, you should think about your achievements and use thatto keep you motivated.

Many people find that dietary supplements and fat burners are also helpful in trying to lose extra pounds. At the moment, there are different kinds of products, ranging from tablets to powders, drinks, and snacks, including cereal bars. These products are designed to do a whole variety of things. Although some might teach you how to burn fat faster, others might show you how to cope with your appetite. Some may show you how to feel fuller and keep full longer, and others may give you an energy boost.

Some products will help your body all at once. For example, a Phen375 product from phen375.com can make it easier to suppress your food drive, boost your metabolism, and increase your energy supply. In general, it can help you to speed up your weight loss, especially when combined with a healthy diet and regular training.

Before you take any kind of dietary aid, you must always seek advice from a doctor who knows your health needs. This is very important because some goods may interfere with the medications or dietary supplements you use, while others may endanger your well-being for several different reasons.

If you want to losea few pounds, make sure you start by tossing out your junk food and eating a healthy and balanced diet. You'll want to receive help from a group to support you, and don't forget to talk to your doctor before you start taking some food products.

IF YOU KNOW THE TRUTH, YOU WILL NEVER LOSE WEIGHT!

Your confidence has more than possibly been shaken by many diet books, slimming pills, and weight-loss strategies that have not succeeded. You will read this before you spend a cent more!

The ways for losing weight are undoubtedly easy.

The real facts researched have shown that carrying the extra pounds is harmful to your health in more than one way. The cause of heart attacks, strokes, high blood pressure, sore joints, chest pains, and digestive disorders is excess weight. I won't continue here, because all this has been read without any doubt before adnauseum, and you know that weight loss means a healthier lifestyle. In addition to looking good, it also means to feel great, more confidence, and a better social life. That is why you want to lose weight as well. It has been shown that by lowering your weight by 5-10%, in general, this reduces the chances of your heart disease or stroke, and your physical health can improve dramatically.

You can't lose weight for real reasons.

A well-known doctor from Arizona has shed light on the real reasons for losing weight in people's digestive systems and colons over several years. The announcement of this recent discovery of why people cannot lose weight has shaken the weight loss industry, and many weight loss consumers have become very dissatisfied with this finding becoming a piece of common knowledge.

This same woman practitioner correctly calculated a conclusive link with persons with chronic obesity between harmful disease and parasite infestations of the human bowel tract. It has been shown that obese people often struggle to achieve a significant loss of weight regardless of the methods of diet.

Your colon produces colonies of up to a hundred different types of parasites with toxins secreted by them, through certain rapid foods and processed foods your store has purchased. These parasites prevent good digestion, and therefore, your weight loss efforts are limited or even fruitless regardless of what you do.

Understanding why you are overweight is the start of real weight loss

Today, a lot of weight loss programs are likely to turn you offand are a total waste of money on the market. This is because these fast paths are useless to lose weight, and some diet plans are unnecessary because they do not use the appropriate criteria for weight loss. In most cases, they are also not good for your health. Fad Diets come and go, and there is a lot of hype in the media. Later, all of this will reduce, and people will be discouraged and disillusioned. If you torture yourself with a weight loss program, it is not for you, and you will probably give up before you lose the pound you want.

Understanding why and where you gained weight is also useful to learn, as that information helps you turn your eating habits into healthy ones.

Weight loss is about diet. Losing weight involves two main activities: regular exercise to burn and cut calories through the choice of intelligent foods and portion control. A one-sided, unbalanced way of creating a calorie deficit is to spend hours in the gym, but it would be impractical and not necessarily fun. Who wants to eat lettuce leaves continuously? Instead, establish these seven easy daily customs to burn fat quickly.

1. Drink eight glasses of water every day. Drink the first thing each morning. The body is more than 60% water and must stay optimally hydrated to operate. We are facing many health challenges, mainly because the body's cells are dehydrated. For starters, we can heal a headache several times by only drinking water. Water holds life's magic. A better understanding of the health benefits of water can alleviate many of the health problems we face in life.

2. Several studies have clearly shown that successful weight loss happens with smaller meals ata regular interval throughout the day and it works for your body. The official recommendation is to have your meals like that and keep them all about the same size.

Smaller meals several times a day were related to more calorie burns after eating, which resulted in better insulin response and lower cholesterol levels in the blood. When you eat regular meals all day long, you will have better control overeating the right portions and less likely to get greedy and overeat.

3. Jumping on a minitrampoline, The National Aeronautics and Space Administration (NASA) has researched the rebounding exercise and found that it is 68 percent more powerful in oxygen than other workouts. What you can tell is that you can exercise intensely without feeling respiratory challenges, and the results are greater than jogging, swimming, cycling, and mountain climbing together. This is excellent news for people who can't play for a variety of reasons. The most significant part of rebounding is enjoyable, and you can skip while watching the news or your favorite TV series.

4. Our wellbeing is directly connected to the way we sleep. Sleep easy. Our quality of life is often said to be linked to our quality of sleep. It is important to be aware that good sleep will contribute to longevity and happiness. Studies have shown that unsuitable sleep can cause a lot of problems and even diseases such as arthritis, insomnia, osteochondrosis, allergy, asthma, radiculitis (inflammatory pain or another discomfort to nerve root), disrupting blood supply and others. The best way to sleep peacefully is to get out of your bedroom all the electronic devices. Create an environment that is quiet, cool, and noiseless with a comfortable mattress. Peace of mind helps to reduce weight effectively.

5. Meditation: life without divine relations is incomplete. Human beings are more than flesh, and we are a threefold being of mind and soul. If we are living our lives without a spiritual connection, we can be angry, depressed, anxious, uncertain, and unsure of the present and the future. A divine relationship can bring life into perspective, and each day makes us face confidence in strength and excitement, all of which can establish a hormonal balance of our system, which improves homeostasis.

Our metabolism is increased then, and weight loss is almost simple during the burning of belly fat. Weight loss is most significant on the waistline, as this is one of the worst places to store excess fat.

Losing weight is very easy if you are committed, thorough, patient, and inspired, of course. There are many solutions to your problems and services that you can join for quick results, as illustrated in the following paragraphs.

The most common solution is to eat less and exercise more often. Nonetheless, there are services and other options you can participate in. Most people die of starvation because they want to losea couple of pounds, but what they do not realize is they are only getting worse because they eat more, and the fat grows in the body.

This helps strengthen the muscles in your body and helps to remove excess fats in the body, thus being the best method to exercise regularly. Exercises such as running, jogging, swimming, cycling are recommended. You may also seek to enroll in an aerobics class;

this does not affect your job; all you have to do is find the right time.

You can also attempt to enroll in a weight loss program. The software helps and promotes you throughout the process. It also helps you keep a healthy food schedule, so you can control the amount of food you eat. It is also recommended that you obey all directions you receive and at the appropriate time.

It is also best to consult the doctor before you begin any procedure because the doctor tells you how much fat you should lose so that it does not damage your body or cause any harm.

Make sure that you get plenty of water every day because it flushes pollution out of your body. In fact, 8-10 cupsof water are suggested.

CHOOSING THE RIGHT WEIGHT LOSS PLAN

Trying to pick a good weight loss plan may be very challenging or complicated if you don't know exactly what to look for in a program. Choosing the right program is a matter of finding an effective program, and it must be one you simply enjoy and comprehend, and it must be easy for you to maintain weight loss guides and techniques.

It is important to choose the right program because it can really mean the difference between success and failure when you lose weight effectively. Finding a great plan is important because it's only half the fight if you lose weight on your own. This is because once you've lost the weight you want, you'd have to learn how to keep it away and an excellent plan will show you how to make it easy.

Now you have chosen to lose weight, how can you choose the right weight loss program to help you to effectively lose weight?

Exhaustion – your baby will often wake up during the night. Try to sleep as much as possible in order to retain your energy levels. Seek to get your baby in rhythm and fall asleep whenyour baby naps. You can both synchronize this and relax while your baby needs you.

Unpredictable schedules and time limits–Seek as far as possible to plan ahead. Find out the eating and sleep habits of your baby and try to work with them. Don't be afraid to ask for assistance, too.

Depression and mood swings – They are easier to handle if you realize that this is natural after childbirth. These symptoms usually go away after a few months. It is good to talk to your partner to support you during this period. Visit your doctor if your postpartum depression or anxiety lasts for a long time or if your family obligations cannot be handled.

Poor Habits – Do not try to lose weight on your own after birth. This is a great opportunity to improve nutrition and health in your life. Get involved with your partner, friend, or loved one. Join a group workout class.

What to do with for exercise?

Seek to include your child in your preparation. You can spend time with your baby and make the training more fun. You can stroll and walk around the city or join the local mommy and me yoga or Pilates.

Break the practice schedules into smaller training sessions that match your schedule. You don't always have to workout constantly. The important thing is that you stay active.

Stay focused–Don't get upset with the time it takes to lose weight with your new child or stress your life. It'll be easier every day as long as you concentrate on yourself and your kids. Be realistic about your goals and be patient.

Fat was created by one dietary supplement and that this dietary addition has no starch, no milk or dairy products, no butter or fat.It was sugar.

This particular fat loss guru told us that we would put in fat stores in proportion to the quantity of sugar in our diets. Many of us already know how mankind in the western world has eaten sugar in increasing amounts at an alarming rate for decades. I understand that the figure now stands at about 50KG per person per year.

My experience was that when I went completely off sugar and strictly limited my fruit use a few years ago, I actually became quite thin for as long as I maintained the diet. As it did not fit with my health awareness or my fruit love for a long time, after several months, I gave this idea away, but it worked and worked very well.

Eliminating all the sugars and most fruit from one's diet can be a great feat beyond the tenacity and bravery of many people, particularly those who love their fruit completely and eat many pieces per day like me or people who cannot take the thought of life without eight cups of tea per day with lots of sugar and scone or cake or muffin.

I've got some great news for you. Method No 2 is this good news. Method 2 is a much simpler, more sustainable, and non-invasive way to lose weight.

An organic network made from amino acids, sugars, and oxygen that serves as molecular antennas for communicating with the human energy field is available today. If this lattice was used, which is programmed like a computer software with the following information, the human energy or magnetic field is programmed. The body cells obtain MAKE ENERGY FAT from the organic grid, and the cells then follow the instructions. Isn't that just right for all of us lazy losers?

It suggests to the fat loser that this pre-programmed organic lattice can be placed on their bodies in the form of patches and worn. It's that easy, actually. The grid interacts with the natural magnetic field of the body, programming the field to use fat to transform it into electricity. All of this, while we go through our normal routine, completely untouched by what the organic grid is for.

Weight Loss Unchained

There are certain rules that don't work as well as their ads. No matter how attractive they sound or how many experts shove the effects of the dedication of subjects on the faces of individuals, such laws must be honestly broken, at least occasionally. After you are aware of the rules that can be broken in your weight loss, you are more likely to lose weight and maintain your target weight.

Here are some thumb rules to follow when it comes to losing weight and weight-in particular when it comes to weight loss. You will ignore anything meant to inspire you to lose weight through intimidation, such as a pair of pants that are too small in many sizes. The reasoning behind this technique is that it will give the subject a feeling of self-insufficiency and thus cause them to work out to try and fit into the clothing. The main disadvantage of this particular method is, however, the adverse always happen; the person finds himself discouraged, irritated, and powerless, a situation that does not make much progress towards achieving his/her goals. Spend anything that doesn't suit. It would also be wise to refrain from weighing yourself every day as you begin to develop muscle regularly; muscle weighs a lot more than fat.

Another weight-loss law that may best help you achieve successis that you insist that all "junk foods" be omitted from your diet. If you delight yourself with the eating of candy, soda, and fast-food products, an immediate cessation of this activity is temporary. The cravings will come back with full force and allow you to dispense in your dissatisfaction with all recent dietary choices. Alternatively, try to circumvent this statute. Reduce the regular intake of calories and keep an eye on what you are consuming but have the luxury of eating fairly unhealthy many days a week, and continue to limit your use of the food until the body feels it no longer needs it.

In fact, if a dietary plan calls for a certain food group to be totally eliminated from your diet, direct attention elsewhere. Proteins are important even if you are a vegetarian. Carbohydrates must be part of your life, even if you decide to commit to the Atkins Diet. You need fats and iron, even if you are overweight. The entire nutrients of your body will work together to properly regulate the functions of your body, and even the loss of a single link in the chain can greatly disrupt your overall health. Be mindful of which foods to eat in moderation and adhere instead to these criteria.

Don't be afraid to be involved in the guidelines/instructions on weight loss. After all, you would prefer to do that rather than risk breaking rules that you don't understand, right? Not all guidelines have positive benefits that accompany a healthy, new lifestyle improvement through weight loss. For more information on which laws are appropriate to be broken, consult your doctor.

You're probably a certain way in some respects. Consider if you go around in circles and face the same problems from time to time. For some women, this is because they choose to have the same sort of routine, and it goes south sooner or later. One example is always trying different diets, different groups, and various weightless workout programs.

do it too. Men do it too. What happens when you have a conversation with someone? Even if you do something like smoking or eating, you will do it ritualistically.

When you eat, you can eat things that are high in fat and sweet. Weightloss isn't about exercise or diet alone. Your emotions control your feelings, causing you to yearn for good, fatty food.

In "thinking," you will be unable to lose weight or meet any other long-term goal that gives you the happiness you desire.

What's the reply?It's the "Be" option.

Of starters, when you lose weight, you have to choose to eat healthily and exercise and keep positive thoughts and images in your mind. This makes you the slimmer person you want to be. You're going to lose weight.

Sounds simple, isn't it? This doesn't seem good, as you know it!

What you can't do is keep these positive thoughts in mind and keep eating unhealthily. If you do, that dream won't stay with you. As you probably are just beginning, you will find that you're very good at eating cake, cookies, pizza, fried things, etc.

Know that sometimes (perhaps often) you're going to blow it. Don't beat yourself up. That just reinforces the idea that you can't do it, which isn't true.

You will choose to be the slimmer person today to achieve this goal in six months or one year. I have great respect for Johann Wolfgang von Goethe, the German philosopher, who said something like this:"Until one is committed, there is hesitancy, the chance to draw back, always ineffectiveness. Concerning all acts of initiative (and creation), there is one elementary truth, the ignorance of which kills countless ideas and splendid plans: that the moment one definitely commits oneself, then Providence moves too."How do you lose weight?

Those who want to lose weight have to understand the fundamental idea behind weight loss. Essentially, it helps to burn fat when the body needs energy and does not get enough of it from the food that you consume. Inorder to lose weight, you must have fewer calories in your daily food intake, as well as having to use the energy that isn't directly available from food. Either one is missing, nothing positive can happen, regardless of what the Internet diet programs tell you.

Clinics for weight loss are killing us!

Weight loss clinics are very risky since most of the healthy things put your body under pressure. There are many deaths caused by such clinics. It is always hidden by covering the death with a concern before the patient went to the doctor. The reasons are profit! All things are about profit and wealth in today's world. The ethically right universe is now only a dream. It no longer exists. It is a good idea to stay away from such clinics.

The best solution: the ultimate weight loss programs offer free trials for at least a week. Trying one of them is worth it because it helps you with your diet, and because you have a trial period, the programs are often very positive. One such software is the dietary supplement for CloudNine Acai Berry. Impressing their customers well is a must because if not, they will lose them. Acai Berry's ability to remove harmful toxins, increase metabolism, increase natural energy, and improve the immune system is established. CloudNine Supplements contain the purest and finest variety of Acai Berries. They help you ease your calorie consumption by suppressing your appetite and clearing your body and provide enough instantaneous energy to exercise.

Some of us are therefore genetically eligible for vegetarian diets, while others are not. Others fulfill nutritional requirements by diet alone, while others require nutritional supplements to alleviate genetic aberration.

If in the cycle of food, we vary in genetics, then we can assume that some of us have an excess of nutrients. Some of us have very low levels of these nutrients, which often cause the RDA to create not a physical but also a mental health imbalance. It is also very important for one to understand that excessive numbers such as copper, iron, folic acid, calcium, and many types of fatty acids may lead to serious health problems as well. This is obviously different from person to person, but multiple vitamins and minerals can damage some and help some.

The scientific studiesagree on the tremendous impact of neurotransmitters on disorder behavior. People can be predisposed to problems because of the genetically aberrant neurotransmitter stage. Our mental health depends on the adequate consumption or presence of nutrients without any essential brain malfunction.

The brain works like a manufacturing company that produces serotonin, dopamine, and different chemicals daily; only the proper consumption of nutrients like vitamins and minerals is the relief for our brain. Improper quantities of nutrients will cause our neurotransmitters to have serious problems. People with depression need basic vitaminB-6 quantities. This vitamin is the nutrient that will synthesize our real suffering in mental health. There are other serotonin-improving drugs and other therapies, but the true cause of mental difficulties still remains uncorrected, so that patients can improvise Vitamin B-6 with supporting nutrients in order to achieve basic health benefits. Thus, nutrient therapy can be extremely potent chemistry without side effects, since no foreign molecules are required to support the body. This approach will potentially remove the need for most psychiatric medications and supervision.

Nutrients have an important role to play in mental health; they are the building blocks of the nervous system, accurate deficiency testing, and comprehension, and overloads can detect many serious psychiatric symptoms and therefore open the way for hope and recuperation.

HOW TO REPLACE YOUR NEGATIVE HABITS AND
EATING PATTERNS WITH POSITIVE ONES

You won't expect to miss your workout once in a while, and then more frequently before you adapt. Usually, this is what happens if you don't have a training plan to follow. Motivation comes from the fact that you benefit.

If you follow a clearly written program that provides constant feedback, you will not need to rely on emotionally-based motivation or control, and all of us know that emotions are desirable.

Doesn't the latest preparation work out? Change is inevitable.

It relates to your wellbeing, nutrition, and athletic objectives more than ever before. If your exercise schedule is too much of a routine, you reach a point of reduction. If you lose interest, you risk injury if you keep going, and most of you will stop looking for help.

Did you reach a plateau during your training? Your body must know that a new program is in operation. Consistent adjustments over a certain period of time give the body a message.

No change will occur if the message is not clear and easy to understand. When the message is clear, easy to understand, and maintained, the body will respond to this shift for a long enough time. Remember, your body is the product of how you live your life every day, with the exception of genetics and environment, of course.

Do you train too much or too little? You can exercise for fitness, weight loss or sport. When you want to have an athletic program when everything you want is to feel better and to work more effectively with painless movement, you'll do too much. Training programming must suit the desired goals and performance, or the outcomes will result in injury, disappointment, or both.

If you aren't a professional athlete who knows well how to research and apply the exercise science for years, you may be able to use some support. Whether you get support from a healthcare professional or from a trustworthy online source, always first seek your doctor's approval.

Over the years, we've seen many diet plans. We also experienced lifestyle plans such as the South Beach diet, the Atkin's diet, fancy exercises, and other high-quality products. The reality still emerged: the diet plans and products that came out very quickly seemed to go away as fast as their rise to fame. This shows that food services are just a good way to get money from the public. Weight loss programs certainly come and go, but perhaps all-diet plans based on one weight loss program stand out.

Mind-based programs are not really food plans or schedules. Such plans are quickly interconnected diet schemes for weight loss. For one way or another, the question is the cause rather than the treatment of the symptoms. These symptoms are the result of eating too much food, which in turn makes us fat because its more than the body needs. If you eat a lot of food, exercise or diet, your minds are solely responsible for all of your actions. In this way, you must understand and learn to control and work your mind for your benefit.

Mind-based programs rely primarily on hypnosis techniques and methods. Hypnosis has been around for so many years, and its effectiveness is quite assured. The software manipulates the mind more or less meaningfully so that you eat less unintentionally. In fact, if you eat a lot, you can eat food that is beneficial to you and you'll lose weight.

What is really important about this program is that it helps you to lose weight without any lifestyle changes. In addition, you can use tailored and quick workout plans to speed up the weight loss process. You must increase your routine with workouts to achieve a really fast weight loss diet plan. You benefit from aerobic exercise, weight-training, and a combination of the two. These exercises will not only make you lose weight more quickly, but they will also strengthen your body. This is because these exercises boost your metabolism, which then gives you more energy to function on a daily basis.

Your Mind Is A Terrible Thing, Just think of it

Why are so many struggling and so few successful? This is not because you're talented or because you have magical powers on your hands. It's just because in their lives something happened that generated a desire to succeed. The loss of weight is nothing other than success. Your mind is the secret to this achievement, and you will be successful until you know that. Failure is brought into the mind even before you start.

To succeed and change the mind, persuading other people is the toughest thing. Why would you like to lose weight? You must have a very good reason to lose weight and achieve the body size that you want. Otherwise, you're going to just fail. What is your reason? Think about it because there the action starts. If your motives to try to accomplish this difficult task are low, you will also have a low chance of success. Ask yourself the question and answer it with conviction.

This example will be serious, but it will help you to understand the way of thinking. Say you met someone who died recently because of some disease caused by their overweight body. Now imagine that this person was your wife, your mom, or your kids. Let us also take for granted that you are overweight and face the same fate. How are you feeling? You have lost a loved one, and now, unless you do something about it, you risk losing yourself. A sense of urgency allows you to persuade yourself to take action and to escape the same fate.

When you find the reason for losing weight and convince your mind that you are going to succeed, the rest is only a walk in the park. You'd overcome the hardest part of any weight loss program. Neve settle for an old lame excuse. Your motives must be strong enough to ensure that your mind doesn't stop.

If you have read anything, I'm sure you read about other people's success stories. In almost each of those stories, you will also notice that they were unhappy, or even suicidal in some extreme cases. Ultimately, reading your stories and finding out why they decided to lose weight will help you to find your own. You're not alone on this trip, so share your stories, and you can share your own success when you succeed.

The body is a machine that is very complex and does its own thing regardless of our intentions. This operates on the following basics: it will tell you when you need food stores that will have surplus food for the future and slows down when you don't have enough food.

Now, look at what you're doing to lose weight.Cut down the food you eat; do more exercise. So, why didn't you try that last time?

Research has shown that the body is sensitive to various situations. By reducing the amount you consume, the body will go into hunger mode. In order to fight it, you can remember feeling exhausted while you were on the last diet. This is your body's way of efficiently using the energy supply, slowing it down. Whatever food you eat is later processed, so you won't only feel tired, but your body won't change shape. Your body will begin to lose muscle definition because it is easier to burn your muscle than fat!

The next time you're at the gym, take this into account. To lose 200 lbs. of fat for a man, he'd have to run at 10mph for 3 hours 20 minutes! If you can run at 10 miles per hour for that long, please send your name and address, the British Olympic Team would like to speak to you!

What is the answer to our objective of intestinal transformation?Try this for 30 days, you won't have a 12-month gym dealor double your food bill for healthy options!

Eat small and often, five meals a day, three hours between meals!

Make breakfast the greatest meal and that your daily consumption. Enjoy your food, take time to chew, stop when you are finished. Nonetheless, follow the rules below.

- Do not eat after 8 pm while you wait 2-3 hours before bed.
- Drink plenty of water (preferably with ice!)
- Get 8 hours ' sleep

This strategy would make your body fat, torment you by starving or over workingyour body in the gym is not important. By adding a few fast building exercises such as press-ups, squats, and sit-ups, it speeds up the metabolism of fat burning.

Most teenagers are dissatisfied with their weight. The more reluctant they are to lose weight, the less effective they sometimes seem. The problem today is how to achieve adolescent weight loss. Understanding the possible causes of adolescent weight problems may help to develop weight-loss strategies for working adolescents.

Heredity definitely plays a role in the form and weight of the body. It is a reality, for example, that different ethnic backgrounds prefer to dispense body fat elsewhere. But that doesn't mean that you are obese just because you have overweight relatives.

Overweight teens must be made aware that given their genes, they can be lean. This is where weight loss programs are put in place for teenagers who prioritize good eating and keeping active.

An overweight parent is behind many an overweight teen. While genes play a role, eating habits learned at home are the most important problem. And don't make a mistake that kids take on their home habits. So if meals often consist of fast food or a bedtime snack is mandatory, don't be surprised when these bad habits are part of the overweight way of life of your teenagers.

It is also important to look at the attitude of the family towards exercise. Should you jump in the car to the convenience store in the corner? Is it your idea ofopening a big bag of chips as the channel flies away? For years, your teen has dealt with this. You're kidding yourself if you think some of these patterns haven't been made theirs.

These are only a few of the causes of adolescent weight problems. The good news is that teen weight loss can only be accomplished if new healthy behaviors are established.

This is a great source for more detailed information on adolescents' weight loss plans.

If your health is at risk, I understand how lucky we are all to have options today, and this revolutionary cold operation will definitely save your life and improve your quality of life dramatically. Yet look at your options and do your research.

However, there is an argument about science. For your details, you need to find an independent source. The problem is that the people who care the most about weight loss surgery are the ones who do it. It would definitely not be in your best interest to advise you against what accounts for the large majority of your profits, and I am not guilty of not focusing on the negative side of this issue. I definitely do not believe something wrong and have great confidence in our overall health care system.

I would like to point you to the only source I have found that is neither prejudiced nor incomplete for quality information. I actually think that this material should be read by anyone who takes some sort of weight loss surgery into account. You must provide this valuable information to yourself and to those who love you. Information that can save your life.

Want to know what to eat and what not to eat? Here are some tips.

1. Eat many fruits! Eat more food! It is a sure way of losing pounds. Try to make every meal part of it. Root vegetables are a great nutrient source, but "pure" vegetables are good for you.

2. Live healthily! Eat smart! The biggest difference between the human being and the beast is the intellect guided by the animal and the instinct. Don't just eat anything you want, be wise, and think about what you'll eat.

3. Pay attention to chocolate and other treats! Most people like chocolates and other forms of sweets, I know, but they're going to add weight. Instead, eat fruit and vegetables. Theytaste good and are much healthier.

4. Try to find set food times. Eat on a regular basis and eat 5-6 times a day. This reduces stress and improves metabolism.

5. Eat when you're hungry! Many of us just eat because we can. Do not do this! Do not do this! You won't get those cravings once you have established a regular eating routine.

6. Stop having snacks between meals. Most people find it difficult to avoid snacking. People who travel a lot also find it difficult to eat properly. However, note that these snacks also contain a lot of sugar, fat, and calories. Instead, try eating berries.

HAS WEIGHT LOSS BECOMES A LOSING BATTLE FOR YOU?

You find it hard, if not impossible, to get rid of these pounds. Have you been exposed to a variety of misunderstandings? Are you ignorant? A little understanding will help you fight your fat. A little bit.

Try these tips to lose weight:

Be not overly enthusiastic: Dieters can often overdo it in combination with excitement and impatience. We can often stop following the recommended diet and take drastic action, such as food avoidance. This will later slow down the metabolism, and therefore, there will be no loss of weight. This reduces the desire and motivation for weight loss. Therefore, always follow the diet map to lose weight.

Schedule your workouts in advance: make arrangements for a certain time and place to do your workout. This will help you keep your appointments and consistently do your workouts.

Morning walks plan: a morning walk gives you a feeling of being healthy all day long because it gives you a feeling that something has been good for you.

Keep a journal: this is a very popular, but valuable point that all dieticians and nutritionists worldwide have listed. Enter all you eat during the day and when. This will allow you to keep a record of what you are consuming and to know where you went wrong, etc. Keeping a diary helps to understand the eating pattern and mood effects on the eating pattern.

Find your personal measures: find out what makes you feel better after a week or two of your diet. Do you like the workouts you have recommended or the diet you follow? If the response is negative, you will change the diet chart and exercise routine to something you want.

Make your diet fun: diet doesn't have to be boring. Make it fun. From ingredients, make new dishes. In addition to eating new things, you will also consume fewer calories.

Find a partner: if you find a friend, it can be more rewarding to go ona diet. It could be a relative or colleague or even your wife, who could also lose weight. In this way, you will enjoy dieting and also learn from the experiences of each other.

Take this expert advice and start again to lose weight. Weight loss can be challenging, but certainly not impossible. But don't give up. You can do it!

Weight Loss Remedy

We avoid our diet because of this: gain more weight and eventually get discouraged. How do you stop making excuses for weight loss?

You make several excuses for losing weight, and it happens naturally without knowing it. Weight loss isn't that easy, but you must control yourself. Next time, ask yourself why every time you tryit, you make excuses.

Some of the most popular reasons are:

- No time to exercise.
- No time to prepare good food.
- Too old to learn. Too old.
- No adequate support or not feeling well.
- Workout is boring.

The above excuses are just a few. You may have found that some of them are just lame excuses. So, how do you stop making excuses for weight loss?

Find out why you are apologizing. Are they acceptable? Or do you know of a better way? If not, why don't you take any action? Some people don't like obesity but don't do it because they are afraid, they will struggle and end up overweight. Don't be scared of change.

How you think will impact how your weight loss routine works. The more you think bad, the more excuses you're going to make and fail. Don't let your low self-esteem triumph over you. Strive harder to find anything important to you.

Lack of time forworkouts is the most common excuse because we're too busy with other things. Time shortage is not a valid excuse, because if we think weight loss is really important to us, we need to find time to do it no matter how busy we are. Practice as much as you can every day, and you will feel more energetic.

To resolve the reasons for weight loss, you must understand why you make an excuse and think about how important it is to you. Discipline yourself, strive to make yourself happy and healthy.

If you have trouble losing weight by yourself, enter support groups where you can meet people who can effectively help you accomplish your weight loss regimen. Clinically proven drugs, including Proactol(TM), a new, clinically proven fat binder, are also available to help you in weight loss issues. It is made of non-soluble and soluble fibers and binds directly to the fat contained in the stomach surface.

It produces a fat-fiber-complex, too large to absorb the fat naturally through the body in the small intestine. Proactol(TM) has been demonstrated to bind up to 28 percent of the dietary fat intake in clinical studies. You should take it after you have eaten. Support groups and drugs such as Proactol help you enjoy a healthier lifestyle.

The weight you lose is just the weight of the body. The loss is temporary and does not contain any fat. Diuretics can cause dangerous dehydration and heart problems. The weight recovers as soon as the body is rehydrated. Significant weight loss includes body fat loss rather than liquids.

One sure way of saying that you are dealing with a diuretic drug is by making outrageous promises, such as "Lose Ten Pounds a Week" or "Lose Ten Pounds in Three Days." You can also see what products are diuretic by looking at the ingredients that are most relevant, according to the FDA.

Caffeine is one of the main culprits. Caffeine can be listed as the main ingredient in a package, or it can be disguised as a green tea ingredient.

Most of the magical formulas of weight loss (in particular those sold as Chinese or miracle teas) contain herbs that act as diuretics.

Only herbs and botanicals, which cause an increase in heart rate, in respiration and other functions do not exist as a "fat-burning herb."

This isn't "fat-burning," it's just tension for the body that can contribute to more calories.

Here is a rundown of some of the most popular herbs mentioned as fat burning or loss of weight, but actually as diuretics.

Buchu. This herb is a strong diuretic native to South Africa.

Dandelion is the safest diuretic and contains two diuretic chemicals, eudesmanolides, and germacranolides, as well as mineral potassium, which contributes to the control of the water balance.

Horse Chestnut. Their main effect is dehydration and symptoms such as dizziness and fatigue. Horse Chestnut is a popular treatment for people with varicose veins and blood pressure problems. It is a strong diuretic that should be used only for one or two days. Dehydration is its main side effect.

Kola Nut. This is a strong diuretic that should not be trivialized. The side effects include prolonged sedation, nervousness, agitation, restlessness, frequent urination, nausea, pain, mania, and insomnia.

Uva Ursi is commonly used in the treatment of bladder infections by increased urine. Neither urination nor dehydration are frequent consequences.

The use of half your body weight of water daily will help your metabolism break down fatty cells and flush out toxins.

If you have a diuretic, think about carbonated sodas and caffeinated drinks. You can cause stomach cramps, nausea, vomiting, or dehydration when taking these forms of supplementary weight loss formulations.

Take 2-3 pounds a week to lose. Yeah, I understand that everyone wants a slim body now, but it's going to have water and muscle and not fat if you lose over 3 pounds.

HOW TO OVERCOME CRAVINGS AND STOP "EMOTIONAL EATING"

QUICK WEIGHT LOSS – CAN IT BE DONE?

Is fast weight loss possible? Not at the pace that everyone would like. A fast loss of weight means loss of as much as 1-2 pounds a week and, if morbid, 3 pounds. Remember that at most, I said. Any plan that encourages 10 pounds to be lost in 10 days cannot be achieved in a healthy way. Such quick-fix strategies also depend on lost water weight, which is recovered as soon as regular diet resumes. Next time you watch an ad on pills like Hydroxycut or TrimSpa, keep your eyes open for fine print that reads something like "Not traditional results." Certain companies use different ways to trick people into thinking that they are the true words of their actual clients. Be wise and don't fall victim to the advertising pseudo-fitness junk; it really is counterproductive.

Myth: Weight Loss Targeting Using Exercises and Products

Another common strategy to be used by people in the telemarketingsector is the endless flood of home fitness devices, which buy a flatter stomach or whatever with three simple payments. Since both men and women are uncertain about their bellies, they are threatened by numerous stand-up and crunchy contraptions in this industry that only encourage minutes of exercise. One of them only encourages 12 repeats on one side and 12 more on the other, giving the owner a well-sculpted set of abs, all within 90 seconds. You can't work in only 90 seconds and expect noticeable results, particularly when you try to isolate one group of muscles in order to cause fat loss. In addition, many fail to realize that ab work leads to stronger abs, not to the subcutaneous loss of weight, which is typically the buyer's target. Don't waste your money on a product that won't give you the results that it boasts.

The best way to lose weight: the perfect way to lose weight is to have a diet where the daily caloric intake is decreased by 500 calories. One could lose a pound of fat a week by simply removing 500 excess calories with diet alone. So drinkyour water and miss dessert instead of drinking two drinks a day and a cookie after lunch. Put this idea together with smaller portions of lean protein and complex carbohydrates and regular meals to avoid hunger pangs. This maintainsthe metabolism so that the body's burning capacity is maximized. As for fitness, work out three days a week and exercise every other day. In fact, ensure that the correct amount of aerobic and anaerobic exercise is integrated. Eat five meals a day, full of colorful fruits and vegetables, lean protein, seeds, and nuts, eat three days a week, and you're sure to lose weight as quickly as your body can!

It can help you understand your body composition, your efforts to gain strength, the activities that are good for you, the foods that help you stay healthy and lose weight, etc.

Genetics will always be a step ahead of them, no matter how difficult some people try. When it comes to fitness or weight loss, you cannot beat your kind of body. Organicfood is an important aspect of fitness, regardless of your body type.

You will improve your health and weight loss by recognizing your body type and learning how to eat to make it become healthy and eliminate any obstacles.

Our body type determines not only how we look but also how our body reacts to the consumption of food. The functions of your hormonal and sympathetic nervous system (SNS) are also determined. It was also established that the type of body of an individual would assess its metabolic capacity and differentiate it from others in the processing of different food types and in gaining or losing weight. It suggests that it is an important factor to maximize your fitness goals.

Most people may look as if they exhibit characteristics of more than one of the following categories, but this is probably due to the years of training and physical care they put into their health and body. Also because of their parents,they could also be a combination of two different body types.Now let's get into what these types of the body mean and what the perfect diet is.

1. Ectomorphic people are slim and strong, which means they have fine limbs and a thin, slender body. The metabolic rates for these

forms are high and are immune to weight gain. But that also means that it is difficult for them to gainmuscles. Ectomorphs can get away from eating large amounts of food without weight gain and have no weight loss issues as well. They have low body fat, of course. But they don't have to workout or live a healthy lifestyle.

What to eat

You should try higher carbohydrates and lower fats if you fall into the ectomorphic group. For this kind, carbohydrates work great. Proteins also have to be ingested in moderate amounts. Fats should be of good quality. Examples include almonds, avocado, chia, extra virgin olive oil and cocoa butter.

Some experts have proposed that the distribution of nutrients in these proportions is optimal for ectomorphs, with 55% carbohydrates, 25% proteins, and 20% fats.

2. Endomorphs often feel that they are the unhappy body. Being one, it often seems to me that we have to work harder than the other two body types to get minimal results.

Endomorphs are often fuller, rounder and appear to store a lot of fat. The form of our body is round and the joints long. We have a big bone structure, and some people often find it a bit more difficult to live an active lifestyle in this group. It may be because of the obstacles and difficulties that they don't want to reach as quickly as they want to be compared with other forms of bodies.

As endomorphs, our metabolic rate is very low, and this helps to store fat and to gain excess weight. For the people with this body, this can be a disincentive and stressful, and it is understandable why some people get fed up and become lazy.

However, that is also not the right answer because once you develop a plan which includes an understanding of your body type, results, and overall success on your weight loss and fitness journey are easier to achieve.

If you know your body type, all the misunderstanding and misconceptions which have made people frustrated will be removed, and things will be easy yet effective. Any diet or regulated food habits will succeed in learning and understanding our body type, in eating for this type of body, and in exercising for this type of body.

What to eat

An endomorphic should consume fats and protein of good quality. As for the consumption of carbohydrates, it is difficult to prioritize healthy fats and proteins while adding some good low-glycemic carbohydrates but is very doable for endomorphs.

Therefore, 25% starch, 35% protein, and 40% fat breakdown. In simple words, it is a great place to start and tweak based on results to consider taking more fats and protein and fewer carbohydrates.

3. Mesomorph, This sort of body, is called genetically talented. Mesomorphs are lean, muscular, competitive, and naturally interested sports. Their bodies are built in proportion and consist of a medium bone structure and a substantially slim waist. People of this type can increase and lose weight easily by changing their diet and level of activity. Mesomorphs can easily build muscle due to high testosterone.

What to eat

You should find a balanced diet if you're a mesomorph. That means dividing the intake of 40% carbohydrates, 30% protein, and 30% fat. You need to concentrate on good weight management throughout your life because you can quickly gain muscle and weight.

We often don't know what our body does for us until it ceases doing it for us. Fitness, weight loss, and wellbeing is easy, but not easy.

Nonetheless, we can make it easier and easier by knowing our body's type. In this way, we get the details, understand the needs, and get the edge to find what we want.

Are you a weight slave?

Should you wake up every morning in fear of getting dressed because you know that your clothes are tight and awkward? You might want to stay with your pants or drawstring pants and skirts that stretch as you do.

You're grumpy and don't understand why, or snap because you're irritated and just can't change.

Does your envy gene come to your attention each time you see a slim person eating a bag of chips that you want and want to do the same?

Is food turning into your nightmare? You are worried about the meals, and you know like you can't eat and drink the same foods as others, and you just feel cheated.

Fear that you have to buy a new outfit, realizing that finding anything that fits or looks good is a struggle once it's done.Our personalities and actions depend on our emotions. If our emotions are out of balance, we become another person to what we were or want to be.

We know we want to lose weight, but we eat comfort food to try and feel better because we're sad. This adds only to our weight problem, and we feel guilty and depressed. The cycle goes round and round.

Diets make us nuts because some foods are removed, and then we crave more, and cheating starts and you know that another diet fails.

Then it's obviously easy to buy ready-made food. It's so easy to stop or get takeout on the way home. This is one of our greatest weaknesses.

There is a remedy, however, but you must be prepared to use it properly.

Rediscover and take control of your body. To do this, you must understand what your body needs to work properly.

Everybody wants to be able to enjoy themselves and go out and do what they want to eat with friends or families. But if you're still obsessed with food and weight, you won't enjoy yourself or envy other people to eat what they want to. You can then order something you won't enjoy or order something you will feel guilty about eating later. You get a better understanding of how you manage your weight by understanding your body and how it uses the food you give it and what is the best way to fuel your body.

You will then understand why you gain weight and lose weight by taking control. Once you understand it, it will be easier to lose weight and regulate your weight.

People don't just eat healthily, but over the years, their conception of portion size has increased even if it is stated that the right portion size is mortifying. "That's not going to support a mouse let me go," they yell.

When have our eating habits and serving sizes changed? When did a meal for fourbecome a meal for one?

There's a preconceived idea that we can't eat enough if the plate isn't packed with food. Much of this is due to suppliers and fast food chains with bigger packaging and great size and all that you can eat buffets.

Therefore, when we are out for a meal, if the serving size is not what is expected, we feel cheated. We only want more at a time. But if you eat more, have larger portions than your body needs and can use, then you'll eventually get bigger.It certainly isn't great!

Food habits and portion size are the secrets to weight control.If your eating habits are bad, your kids have a good chance of eating like that too.

In Britain, healthy food is added to school meals, and nutrition is considered part of the curriculum. Teaching children to eat properly will eventually lead to healthy adults. We hope to counter the epidemic of obesity through education.

Allow children to eat healthily so that they don't want unhealthy food.One way to help is to provide your child with interesting and simple food as a parent or guardian. Most schools have time to eat so that the meal is simple for children.

It may be mentioned that hard-boiled eggs, proper cheese bits, raisins, vegetable sticks, and already sliced vegetables, crackers, or cereal may be easier to eat and more appealing.Healthy food must not be boring or even unpleasant. It doesn't have to take time to prepare healthy foods either.

With the issue of diabetes and obesity currently at the forefront, most restaurants and even fast food outlets offer a healthier choice. It is up to you, though, to make the decisions.

A good understanding of how the body uses food help to encourage weight loss. People get caught up in the consumption of calories but do not really know what is best for them. Some assume you can never again have a sweet, but that doesn't have to be the case.

Do we really understand what the different types are when we talk about food? For example, do you think this food is good for the body as it provides energy when you think of potatoes? Or are you sure you're just going to gainweight? Pumpkin is the carbohydrate, and we need energy carbs. But the trick to eat carbohydrates is not what but how much. This is why it is so important to have a portion size.

Knowing the body and knowing the right size is the secret to weight control. Too much food can contribute to too much of you because your body can use only so much food at once. Therefore, you need to understand the needs of your body before you begin to lose weight.

You will first need to calculate and weigh your portions to see what is right for you. Smaller portions of carbohydrates and proteins and more vegetables are required. After a while, it is easy and natural to take only the right quantities.

If you can afford it, you can get rid of your big plates and bowls and replace them with a smaller one. Your plate doesn't look half full, so you won't feel robbed.

Eat slowly, let your body have time to know that it is fed and will alter your system of hunger and satisfy you. If you eat quickly, then later, you feel uncomfortably full.

Know what foods are right for you, and eat what you like, instead of pushing you to have things that you don't like. Know what foods should not be consumed regularly, so you and your family can see them as special treats.

Make food a sociable moment, so you can look forward to it and feel better. Remember not to get so hungry you're just eating anything. Think ahead, always have some fruit, vegetables, or a healthy snack bar in your bag or office instead of eating a meal.

If in restaurants you have to eat a lot, make healthy choices. When you order your meal, ask for sauce or dressings on your side. You are in charge in this way. Request a greater amount of vegetables and fewer carbohydrates. Select leaner or even better red meat cuts, select chicken or fish dishes. When the bread is delivered before the meal, put a piece on your side dish, instead of filling it up, and then force yourself to eat. Share a starter instead of having the whole thing, if possible.

When people try hardest to lose weight

So many people say they tried everything to conserve these unwanted pounds, but their efforts were clearly not enough. If you fail in your weight loss plans, it is usually because of your own lack of control.

The first part of your weight loss plans is to get rid of the quick fixes that supplements and pills promise and start with the proper diet and exercise schedule. Although experts constantly tell us that the right diet and work out are the solution to the weight problem of all, it is also well known that not everyone has benefited completely. There is a simple fix for those who have tried and failed in weight loss programs. What we have to do is find the right plan and our lifestyle.

To meet the weight loss objectives is to take steps and recognize that it takes time to achieve those goals by taking themstep by step. Many people fail because they expect their lives to turn around overnight rather than realizing that it takes time to achieve the desired results. You need at least two weeks to make a change in your lifestyle to become part of your normal and everyday habit. To actually do this, your lifestyle takes far more time to fully incorporate with who you are.

When it comes to your weight loss, it is important to stick to the program that you choose and do not cheat very often. One simple step that many people find not only helpful is to eat more fruits and vegetables and to stay away from fast foods and foods full of fat. Many people try to go directly to the diet of raw food, but most people can't. You have to consider your own limits when determining which steps you will take to achieve your weight loss goals. You certainly want to do this step by step on the basis of these weaknesses instead of startling the mechanism by sudden actions that lead to failure.

Some people who use the raw food diet claim they get all the nutrients they need from the food. You may find that some of the people who have taken their rough diet over the months have become healthier. It should not be shocking that not everyone has self-control over a long period of time to eat raw food. But if you decide to give it a try and have the courage to stick with it, then give it a shot by all means. There are various sites on the Internet for a raw food diet. I would suggest you review so that you have the greatest chance of success.

You should now realize that you have self-control and discipline while you adopt a diet. Self-control requires the ability to understand our goals and take the necessary steps to ensure we comply with our weight loss and diet plan.

Although it has been said on several occasions that a good workout scheme following your healthy diet will help improve the level of fat loss and trimming. Exercise increases the metabolism of the body, and the workout will pump your blood, and your system will purify your sweat with toxins. Such benefits of exercise allow you to stay healthy and in the best way possible.

Another thing to do to accomplish your objectives is to drink water, which is often overlooked. By drinking water, you will often feel full and, therefore, less likely to binge and also recover missing fluids from your perspiration. You will also need water to support your internal organs. The experts advise that every person should drink between 8 and 10 glasses of water every day. However, other medical professionals may handle this differently, depending on the medical condition of the individual. The benefit of drinking water is also to increase our metabolism and to minimize body fat by burning calories.

When it comes to your weight loss plans, when you stick to the plan that suits you and takes plenty of water into account, you'll find yourself slowly progressing. But you need self-control in order to stay with it long enough.

The most important thing to remember is self-control. You can only act and continue until this is part of your lifestyle, which provides long-term benefits.

CONCLUSION

WAYS TO HELP YOU LOSE WEIGHT

To get rid of extra fat, one needs to incorporate total simplicity and exercise science because it helps to understand how to get rid of body fat. You can now make your body look like you want it and fulfill your long-lasting vision of losing extra fat.

As soon as you find out the solution to losing weight' properly, you are on the right path to fitness. So, it's a simple matter to get rid of extra fat. Yeah, of course, in your preliminary opinion, the trouble you might face may hinder you from starting.

There are many things you will have to do to get rid of extra fat. If you're willing and ready to do this, you'll get rid of extra fat.

After you have basically reprogrammed yourself completely on weight loss by seeking tools that do not really understand the truth, or even worse, just try to do what you need to detach from the checkbook, charging card, or even the pocketbook — the actual simple and long-term duality of the way to get rid of additional fat is uncontrolled.

Someone (that means you) has to do the job! You want to get rid of extra fat, that's precisely why you're here. Therefore, the body has to participate in time-proven, expert ideas that confirm more than just once for you. In short, to lose body fat, you are clearly building freedom, trust, and other losing-body fat skills that emanate remarkably from your psychological, intellectual potential rather than just your current abilities.

The three steps towards weight loss are right here:

First: once and for all, learn to figure out how to use your calories and how they affect energy levels. Those two proportions are typically important to your general health, so that you know exactly what your body does, all the way to the single calorie.

Second: typically work out using much more energy and power than you have ever had before in your entire life! This is only because 1) far from other people who have conscious human behaviors; everyone has to take a rest and use the easiest way out of a difficult situation, rather than facing it and overcoming itstrue cause. However, 2) recommended fitness science tells you that workouts at a higher level prolong your lifespan and burnmore calories. Therefore, to lose huge but proper body fat, start teaching yourself to work out for prolonged intensity.

Thirdly, remember that the entire situation circles around 1, which is both necessary and unchanging: obesity, thus, having to lose extra fat, remains a direct result of eating too much food and having not enough workouts. The issue is that the person listens very much to theloser system, unwanted fat knowledge, and thus often that the human brain instantly retreats into sleep or even shuts off. Knowing the true significance of what needs to be done to get rid of body fat involves visibility, accessible mind, and motion.

Who makes you fat, and how do you avoid it?

The true, bad news, as most of you already know, is that fat doesn't make you obese but carbohydrates high in sugar can result in a corresponding increase in weight. What is the connection between exercise and nutrition for weight loss and weight maintenance? As you age, there is a chance of raising your need for exercise to burn more calories.

Excessive exercise during your later years has an effect on the body that is related to stress and contributes to catabolic (muscle breakdown) disease.

If you want to lose weight, a viable option remains, eat fewer foods via portion control. Although not a new concept, this is still one of the most daunting behaviors. There are a number of reasons why people overeat. The most convincing is the role emotions play in the consumption of food.

Stop getting fat. Think about a distressing event that happened recently in your life? It could have been related to work or school. What have you done to prepare yourself for the event? I'm sure many people nod their heads and accept their food as a means of comfort.

Emotions play a key role in your health management during stressful times. You usually understand how good food can be during these times. So, what are you looking for? It is definitely likely that throughout your life, you will face stress-related situations.

This is why it is important that you understand how to direct yourself through the dangers of getting entangled in your emotions.

My plan is as follows. Pay attention when you snack. It is important to avoid distractions in your environment, as this prevents your connection with your food. I speak of being mindful of how much food you put into your mouth during meals when I talk of this link.

When you see TV when you eat, you tend to focus on the show you watch and less on the food in front of you. Your mind wanders; when you sleep, you go into an unconscious state. You're more likely to overeat when you ignore the cues that your body transmits. Being present ensures that you are accustomed to the signs and feelings of your body. This is called an interception.

The other important strategy is to take feelings into account. Do not eat while upset. Read that sentence again and bring it into memory. It is important that you understand the emotional reaction process of your body. Understanding your mental constitution helps you to navigate your way out of over-alimentation. Understanding the behavior patterns in order to change it is a valuable long-term success technique.

My advice is not to transform food into emotional turmoil to comfort. That is why I promote and write articles. This empowers people to understand their emotions in order to improve themselves.

You become alert and wake up to many circumstances in which life presents you. You stay calm and still in turbulent times because the experience of your outer world does not affect your inner world.

Your awareness and your body relationship is a journey. Part of this trip means that you will inevitably choose the wrong route. You don't have to fear that you have lost your way. You simply learn what you can't do on a path that involves multiple detours.

Stay calm and well-balanced in difficult times. Know your faults. Stay aware of things that work and not. In a short time, you will be armed with the knowledge to follow your goals in a body that radiates diverse health and vitality.

Lastly, self-hypnosis for weight-loss is pretty easy to practice. You utilize methods such as visualization and favorable self-talk to configure your mind to believe in a new way after you have actually brought your body into a totally unwinded state.

ACTION 1

The very first thing you require to do to practice self-hypnosis for weight loss is to get comfy. To release stress in your body start by tensing then relaxing each part of your body beginning from your forehead down to your toes.

ACTION 2

As you gradually exhale repeat the word unwind to yourself. To deepen your sense of relaxation, you can envision yourself going down a long flight of stairs slowly or just count down from 100 as you focus on your body unwinding more and more.

STEP 3

When you are totally relaxed, you will use positive affirmations to deal with the concerns concerning you. If you're using self-hypnosis for weight reduction, you may want to attempt suggestions like "I delight in the taste of vegetables and fruit," "I like how I feel after I exercise,"or "I take pleasure in being slim and fit." You're simply required to keep repeating these affirmations until you feel satisfied.

ACTION 4

To come back to awareness just count from 0 to 10 while focusing on the numbers until you feel completely awake. You might have to count from 0 to 10 more than once until you feel prepared to get up and begin normal activities once again.

Developing your own self-hypnosis for weight-loss program will go a long way to helping you finally conquer the obstacles holding you back from losing weight and keeping it off.

Do Not Go Yet; One Last Thing to Do

If you enjoyed this book or found it useful, I would be very grateful if you would post a short review on Amazon. Your support does make a difference, and I read all the reviews personally so I can get your feedback and make this book even better.

Thanks again for your support!

CPSIA information can be obtained
at www.ICGtesting.com
Printed in the USA
BVHW041044110321
602311BV00004B/228